REVIEWS

Being brought up in Al-Anon and losing my son to a drug overdose, I did not think there was much to learn about addiction that I did not already know. The spiritual aspect of addiction as told by Jay changed everything for me in how I view its cause and its remedy. Prime Threat – Shattering the Power of Addictions shares principals that are a guide to life, not just new guidelines for addiction. Once again, Joan Peck brings much needed *soul*utions to our awareness. Yes, we can live without addiction.

Regina Murphy,
Author - "The Elusive Gift of Tragedy"
Founder of "Emotional Sound Techniques"

Prime Threat – Shattering the Power of Addiction is utterly fascinating, thought provoking, and full of exciting possibilities. It is a stimulating and comforting book which reveals the path to overcoming addictions. It is both insightful and informative.

If you read it with an open mind, you will find it to be tremendously helpful to you in learning how to develop the inner strength to live a life of peace and purpose: a life that is rich, joyful, and meaningful no matter what is happening on the outside. The author, Joan Peck, understands and appreciates life at a higher level.

Judi Moreo
Author – "You Are More Than Enough"

So many of us who have returned to help heal the negativity on Earth are delighted when a book such as Prime Threat – Shattering the Power of

Addiction becomes available. It is a book that lovingly shares channeled conversations between a mother and her son who died due to his addictions, answering many of the questions any of us who have lost a loved one to addiction wants to know. Open your mind and heart as you read this book and rejoice in all the possibilities that life has to offer knowing it is up to each of us how we choose to live. Let Prime Threat show you the way to live without destructive addiction and live one filled with love, joy and gratitude for being here.

Doreen Ping
Author – "Stretching Beyond Life's Boundaries" Intuitive Counselor

PRIME THREAT

SHATTERING THE POWER OF ADDICTION

BY JOAN S. PECK

Published by Bejeweled Publishing

6480 Annie Oakley Dr. #513
Las Vegas, NV 89120

Manufactured in the United States of America.

ISBN: 978-0-9824607-7-1

CONTENTS

LEARN TO LOVE AND ALL ADDICTION WILL CEASE

NEXT TIME, I WILL . . .

In another time, and place
I would change my forever
Run in the wind
Forget my pain altogether.

I'd walk in the valley
Of the future and the past
Staying only in the moments
That I want to last.

I'd dance in the rain
Allow for my moment to soar
Remove fear of resistance
For ever more.

I'd gather my pieces
Build my desire from there
Remove unknowing sorrow
Release the despair.

I'd hold on without a
Chance to ever withdraw
Taking with me always
The unending love I recall.

I'd stand in the light
Revealing what I lost
Give up my doubt
No matter what it cost.

I'd explain to myself
What all means to me,
Savor every moment,
  The chance to be free.

I'd shine in the joy,
Let my essence pour through
Continuing on my journey,
Embracing what is new.

I'd live out my dreams
I would not hold back,
Believe in why I am here
Never getting off track.

I'd allow for the strangeness
And the chance to explore
Learn who I'm becoming
Never fighting it anymore.

I'd scream out
What I am holding within
And allow for the magic
To never end.

I'd live for today,
Leaving nothing undone
Giving myself forever
To finish what I've begun.

Donna Vicchiullo, 2011

DEDICATION

This book is dedicated to each and every one of us here on the earth plane and those beyond the veil. Each is the other - all One. May we recognize that in order to survive on this planet (or any other), we have the responsibility to simply love each other and allow the space for each individual's journey in life. There is too much anger and hate in the world today. It is time to love and honor each other so that we are able to assist those who need our help, especially those children coming in who are hoping to face and clear their addictions. Breathe in the possibility of Oneness; breathe out the love in your heart to all those in need of it. You will change the world! Believe it!

ACKNOWLEDGMENTS

Jay and I acknowledge all the souls who have supported us on our own journey of discovery and healing – all the Masters, Guides, Angels and Spirits, and those individuals here on earth who have aided us along the way. We are grateful that with your help, we have the opportunity to share some of what we have learned about addictions in the hope that it helps others. Love and light to you all.

Thank you, John Perotti. You have been a blessing in my life, and I am grateful for having you be part of it.

Thank you, Cheryl Johnson, dear heart, for all your love and the power of your channeling Jay and the others. It has been a fun "ride" for both of us – one that I will forever be grateful.

Thank you to my friend, Donna Vicchiullo, who so lovingly gave me the poem she had written to be a part of this book. You are a beautiful poet and soul.

Thank you dear family and friends who have encouraged me and supported me in this endeavor: my dear friends, Doreen Ping, Ann Frazier, Karen Coltin, Anne Heim, Darlene Navarre, Gulten Dye, Jeannine Mason, and the list goes on - too many to name. You know who you are, and I am blessed to have you in my life. Please know that I love and honor you.

Thank you, Regina Murphy, who so graciously gives of her time and wisdom to help others. Your work will know no limits as the world comes to recognize your efforts and the power of sound to heal. We are grateful for the information that you share with us.

I personally thank my three children for all that we have shared together in life – the good and the more difficult. I am proud that you chose me as your mother this lifetime and allowed me to muddle through it. Jen and Shelly, I am so very proud of you both. You are beautiful souls with much wisdom to offer others, much of which will help to keep others on the straight and narrow – and loved. Jay, I know your heart in ways hard to describe. I am so very proud of you for wanting to share your experiences, what you have learned and what you are doing to connect again with who you really are as part of all that is, a beautiful soul. Thank you, my children, from my heart where you will always reside. I love you completely.

PREFACE

My son, Jay, died of a drug overdose in 2005. He was 36. It had been a long battle throughout the years where he was in and out of rehab many times. Always struggling with his addiction, he sought drugs again after a time of being sober and clean.

In the later years when my son's addiction was the strongest, an atmosphere of "waiting for the other shoe to drop" was created and hung over the heads of all that were near - family, friends or acquaintances. Remember, *we all get to ride the pony with the one that is addicted whether we want to or not.*

Toward the end of Jay's life, living became unbearable for him. He was physically ill and the addictions had become so severe that any chance of recovery became slimmer and slimmer.

But the truth is that I have known since Jay was a small child that he would not outlive me. No one said anything out loud; there were no words spoken. It was just something I knew and it made me cling to him a bit more in silent defiance against the inevitable. I have spoken to other parents who have lost a child to addiction and many of them, too, have had a sense from young childhood that their child would have an early death.

I love Jay and miss seeing him in person every day. We had been close in life and it was hard to let him go. I wished, pleaded and begged for a different ending for him. But was his ending really what was meant to be?

I have learned through time and experience and the simple belief in God that we are here on this earth plane to experience life. For each of us that is different. If you believe as I do, we choose our parents, family members and what issues we want to deal with in life as a learning experience so that we may experience ALL of life. That means that happenings, including addiction, may be something the addict has chosen to work on and hopefully clear.

My belief is that for this lifetime, Jay and I agreed to be mother and son. He would come in with addictions and the deal was that he would either kick his addictions and we would share some information regarding what we had learned or he would die before me and we would work together (he from the other side) to share what we have learned about addictions and to help those dealing with it.

I thought that I knew all I wanted to know about addiction to last a lifetime. What a laugh! I only knew what I knew through limited resources and riding the coattails of my son's addictions without delving into the complete understanding of addiction. I guess I had been in "survivor" mode. After Jay's death, I learned that his life and what we are doing has meaning far beyond what I had thought. And this book is a part of that.

I met Cheryl Johnson shortly after Jay's death and she channeled him in so that I could ask some questions and thank him for some information he had sent me where he reminded me not to own other people's negative reactions and comments concerning his death.

I connected with Cheryl right away, for she is an amazing woman and soul filled with insight, love, light, and humor. When I sit with her and watch her reactions to some of Jay's thoughts and humor, she is much like the proud mother. What a humbling experience to realize that she is as much a mother to him as I was when I showed him love, tolerance, non-judgment and acceptance. Cheryl reminds me time and again how we are all connected ... all one ... on an awesome journey of experiences.

As I spoke with Cheryl and worked through some of my sorrow, I began to understand that I had a commitment to my son to complete our pre-lifetime agreement. I became determined to do so; yet, there was so much for me to learn! I began with understanding in greater depth the seven major chakras and their energies and wrote two books about them. My third book is an anthology of 28 different spiritual modalities which is unique serving more like an encyclopedia. By doing this, it gave me time to grow spiritually and to really understand that ALL (every single thing!) is ENERGY. That is the **key** to understanding ourselves; what and who we bring into our lives, and the ability to heal ourselves.

In this book, we discuss Jay's addictions, which gives us greater understanding of what they are and how we develop addiction and even bring them forth through lifetimes. I need to be clear though ... *we all have addictions even if you think you don't*. A thought and a belief that is negative or untrue that we own and hold captive can be as caustic in its own way as many of those destructive behaviors that belong to the addicted of drugs, alcohol, gambling, sex, shopping, cutting one's self, plastic surgery, internet games, base jumping, food, and many more and all other addictions. Many times they are just not as showy in its damage. But they are there.

Besides fulfilling our pre-lifetime contract, this book was written by us to assist and guide those who are looking for greater understanding of addiction and for a way to live *without* addiction. If you have picked this book up to read, it is no coincidence that you have. As you read on, you will become aware that you have a role to play in healing addictions within our societies from this minute forward.

By reading this book, you are prepared to reach out and help others that are already here or those who are coming to us now and will be coming to us in the future who need your love and understanding of *how to shatter the power of addictions*, addictions being the Prime Threat of remaining in the lower energy dimensions where negativity, judgment and lack of love has a greater chance to survive.

If we are to eliminate addictions and create a healthier, happier existence for all, it begins with understanding addiction and how it plays out in our own living. It includes having the courage to look at and change any of our own negative beliefs about addiction so that we can help those with destructive addictions face them and clear them. *We are their hope.* And your reward is the knowing when you share your light of goodness with others, you find your authentic self. This is a divine gift in itself.

Cheryl, Jay and the "Others," and I have joined together to share with you what we know and have learned about addiction. Going forward in this book, for simplicity sake, we will refer our collective thoughts as through "Jay." Just to be clear, there is in addition to Jay, a group of souls on the other side that we sit with in our discussions who are friends, guides, Masters and angels - all part of our agreement to share with you our knowledge about addiction. It is our hope that we can help all who are addicted begin to heal and live healthier lives. Understanding addiction and how best to cope with it and let it go gives us hope and lightness to look forward to the future, living in healthy ways. And it helps us make better choices.

We meet Jay and look at addiction from a greater spiritual side via some of Jay's personal lifetimes. We will delve deeper into the effects of past lives, DNA and cellular memory, all of which has the ability to bring forth a need that seemingly can only be satisfied by its addiction to whatever creates the satisfaction of that need. We will embrace changing our perspective from "omit" to "replace," and free ourselves from addiction through the understanding that the free flow of energy brings us to the highest vibration (replacing anything of lower vibration) connecting us to Source. In other words, we can be addiction free. *Yes, it is possible.*

Let me explain what I mean when I say "replace" our addictions. Nothing replaces addiction in the sense that once we experience the "high" of any addiction and the euphoria that comes with it, there is no "replacement" for it. For example, how do you replace the euphoria and ultimate high reached when you inject or swallow a drug? The experience is what it is - for any addiction. However, you can **"incorporate"** the memory of the good feelings or the "high" of your addiction into everyday living. You **"replace"** what the body, mind and spirit has already experienced in the addiction high into your quest for spiritual living. You can bring up to a lesser degree that same euphoric feeling and incorporate it into even the smallest experiences in life – watching a bird build a nest or washing your hands. It takes time and practice, but the end result is worth the effort. It is like anything else – the more you do it, the easier it becomes.

What we share with you is how you can get into that space of understanding, and the ultimate knowing and belief of who you truly are as part of All That Is. That is when you are able to release yourself from trying to control your life and escape from it. That is when you learn the difference between what you can control and what you can't. That is when you have acceptance that all is as it should be according to what *you have created*. That is when you are able to get to the seat of your addiction and have it in front of you so you can begin to *clear* that aspect of fear. That is when it is your own CHOICE and not something you have to do for someone else or simply because you have been forced to do it. It is when you understand that you choose the life you want to lead and have the *power* to do so. That is when you start living your power in joy and peace.

We look at the different steps and formulas for *living **without** addiction now*. There are ways and routines to change your addicted way of living to one of fulfillment without the downward spiral of any disease behavior that doesn't serve you. We look at living life from the "inner knowings" that exist in each of us - living to our highest good and the highest good of all and extending that to live fully and completely in our outward-focused society. We present a clearer understanding of how energy works, and how to create positive energies, particularly the love energy - the highest vibration. We look at vibrational frequencies and learn how to use them to heal many different issues.

When you read what Jay has to say, we hope that you will feel as we did – filled with hope, peace, and a greater appreciation for what they have shared with us and the experience of living at this time on the earth plane when there is so much positive change in the works.

Jay gives us a greater understanding of energy and we become even more familiar with the energies of the 7 major chakras as they relate them to addiction in a more futuristic sense. Then, lastly, we look at the God energy to clarify what it is and why we would even choose to be here on earth in human form. As always, what they say is fascinating.

You are invited into our sessions where our discussion sometimes has a "life of its own" when we go from one thought to another. But as you relax and join us in the sessions, you will simply become caught up in what we are saying and all will become clear. Just open your heart and mind and take from our discussions what makes sense to you. Let go of any judgments and let life flow easier for you with the acceptance that love in all positive ways cures all and is our purpose for living. Understand that love begins with self.

Whether you are the addict or the one living or involved with one, the hardest thing to do is to open up to really look at all aspects of *yourself* - to recognize your own past choices, thoughts, prejudices, judgments and all the rest; have the strength and courage to forgive yourself and others, and *let it all go*. When you are able to do so, this leaves you with the love of the Divine that moves you ahead in a positive, healthy way.

But no one said that life was for the weak. So hang on … here we go.

OUR SPIRITUAL PHILOSOPHY

A dear friend suggested that if we would be willing to share with you, our readers, our spiritual philosophy, you would have an even greater appreciation of this book and all the wondrous news that Jay is giving us. We enthusiastically agreed and are happy to present our "truth" to you.

We believe that each of us has our own energy that was first created by whatever name you desire to call your higher power – God, Goddess, Source, The Universe, Allah, Intellectual Intelligence and so forth – plus the experiences you have had through lifetimes of living. These experiences make up your "filter" of processing happenings and the way you think about things. It is those different lifetimes and events that make each of us unique for no two people experience the exact same thing all the time.

Yet, because we all are birthed from the same energy of the Creator, we are and always will be ONE energy in spite of our different lifetimes and experiences. In other words, because of the energy of one that exists in each of us, what one of us thinks about or acts on, affects the rest of us even if only in miniscule ways. That thought, word or action that we have is a movement of energy holding a vibration, whether higher or lower, that has either a positive or negative effect in the energy of one. This works the same way for each of us with no deference to color, race, creeds or anything else. Basically, we are all the same within our soul (original) energy; yet, we are very powerful as individuals! We are creating all the time, every moment, with each thought, word or action. How we can use our positive energy or change any negative energy we have created is what Jay is sharing with us through his own experiences! Yes, we can choose the life we want to live! There is hope for us all to live the best life possible!

Let us explain in a very simplistic way how the effect of an individual's energy works in relationship to the one energy:

Let's pretend that each of us on earth is an apple, each one special and unique because we know that no two people carry the same experiences with them. My apple is different from your apple, yours is different from mine or anyone else's, etc.

Now, let's pool together all the apples here on earth and make a big pot of applesauce. As all of those apples are joined together, it is hard to differentiate one individual apple from another, isn't it?

Since each apple has its own energy of thoughts, words and actions, just one single apple has great *power* to change the entire pot of applesauce. If you can envision the applesauce as the energy of one, and watch as one of the apples within the applesauce increases its energy of thoughts, words, and actions to the highest energy of love, what happens to the applesauce? It becomes sweeter, affecting all the other apples! Each individual has the power to change the energy of the one, whether positive or negative. Amazing, isn't it?

In addition, we also believe that it is a privilege to be here as a human being at this time on earth where many of us have agreed to share with others more of the spiritual way of living, lightening the load of the heavier 3rd dimension, moving us forward to the 4th and 5th dimensions. This enables the more positive effect of the energy of love, the highest dimension. Just so you know, not all of us are doing this by writing a book or conducting a seminar or otherwise. Some are simply modeling for others loving behavior in everyday life. It is at this level of love that we can truly enjoy what earth was created for - a special place where there is acceptance of each other without judgment. A place where we are willing to care for and marvel in all the magnificence and beauty that Mother Nature provides with its animals, insects, fauna and more. A place where it is recognized that each person has his or her own journey and we are there to simply encourage and support them, nothing else. A place that knows no boundary in unconditional love. Only then will this become a place of true enlightenment, a nirvana.

Throughout our story, we have used words in a spiritual sense that are also used and identified in more traditional ways. This may cause you some confusion and block clear understanding and the significance of what is really *exciting news* coming from Jay, who is gaining knowledge about his own addictions and is willing to share what he is learning with us. We have simplified some of the basic terms that we easily discuss throughout the book: frequency, vibrations, and dimensions - which all has to do with energy. Since everything is energy and is always moving – just at different speeds – and is always created by each of us, here is how we define those terms compared to how they show up in a dictionary:

Definition: Frequency is the rate at which a vibration occurs that constitutes a wave, either in a material (as in sound waves), or in an electromagnetic field (as in radio waves and light), usually measured per second.

Spiritually, we use the term frequency to denote the degree of vibration (higher or lower) that we have created and surrounds our body.

Definition: Vibration is an oscillation of the parts of a fluid or an elastic solid whose equilibrium has been disturbed, or of an electromagnetic wave.

Spiritually, we use the term vibration as a person's emotional state, the atmosphere of a place, or the associations of an object, as communicated to and felt by others.

Definition: Dimension is an aspect or feature of a situation, problem, or thing; a measurable extent of some kind, such as length, breadth, depth or height.

Spiritually - in the spiritual dimension, negative energy is lower vibration because it is denser and heavier. Positive energy is higher vibration because it is finer and lighter. This relates to the added belief that all negative energy makes you feel trapped and heavy; all positive energy makes you feel free and light. That is the difference between joy and grief, peace and stress, clarity and frustration. And we each have control over this!

When we talk about enlightenment, it is that aspect of spiritual growth that is willing to let go of negative thoughts, words and action and connects us more closely with our higher power (which we call God), living life with the purity of our soul energy that we had when we were first created. We refer to that purity as "light."

In our book, we also speak of Jesus, the Masters, Angels and Ancient Ones as being in the higher dimensions and are those energies and spirits who in simple terms have had more experiences living in the light. Some choose to return to earth from time to time to live as teachers without recognition, who have come back for all different reasons. They can be the stranger who acts in small ways to help you when you are lost, or the one who smiles at you when you are down or the beggar on the street, reminding you to share with the less fortunate. One never knows. The Universe is always providing for us – we just have to be aware of all the signs, messages and signals sent to us. Life is good. Just open your heart to all its goodness.

With all of this being said, we hope that these pages help you better understand what lies ahead for you as you peruse our story and begin to absorb all the glorious and magnificent information that Jay shares with us. Open your mind and heart knowing that we send you blessings and light as you read along.

Introduction

What is addiction?

When you hear the word *Addiction* or *Addict*, what is the first thing that comes to mind? How does the word make you feel? Does it cause a flutter in your stomach? Do you immediately think of someone you know that is addicted or do you worry that *you* might be the addict? Do you feel loss because someone you know has lost their life to addiction? Do you blame yourself or others for that loss?

With one out of every three people affected by drug or alcohol addiction either by being an addict or close to someone who is just hearing the word addiction can cause a sinking feeling in the pit of our stomach. And sometimes, that feeling can remain with us for a long time.

Many times we can be caught off-guard when addiction becomes a reality in our lives. I remember when I was first told (nearly 45 years ago) that my ex-husband was actually an alcoholic and not just someone enjoying a "few beers" socially each day. I had no idea really what that involved or why my husband was the way he was. Our relationship was not in a healthy place and without understanding addiction, I had no way to separate his behavior into the different slots of addictive behavior, mental illness, bad manners or other behavioral issues that were making our entire family miserable. Nor did I know what to do with it! And something I wouldn't address until later in my life was any thought as to what, if any, my role might have been in it.

At that time, we didn't have all the information available to us that is at our finger tips today and my understanding of what was really going on was limited. It is only by trying to understand what my family was going through then and years later, and attending a few AA and Al-anon meetings, and reading some of the materials available that I was able to glean anything about addiction (remember we didn't have the internet then). And yet, I still wasn't understanding addiction on a deeper level until Jay and I, with Cheryl Johnson delved into it on a spiritual level.

I wish that I had this information presented here years ago. What is that expression? "if wishes were horses, beggars would ride" . . . Would it have changed things? I don't know . . . but I have to believe it would have.

So with the belief that Jay's and my life purpose is to assist others in learning about addiction, we write these chapters to give you as clear an understanding as possible of what addiction is, how it works and its effects.

I have learned so much about addiction and life itself since Jay's death in 2005 that at times all the years previous to then seem to have been the long way home. Our hope is that what we share with you will help ease your own way through life, discovering your own power to create a life filled with love and light.

WHAT IS ADDICTION?

Before you can understand why an individual develops an addiction, you must cultivate a basic understanding of the affliction's core definition. Addiction is defined by the medical field as something which produces a physical and psychological need within the sufferer.

Although we could simplify the definition by stating that an addiction is simply satisfying a need no matter the consequences, it is so much more than that ....

What is that need? Simply put, we get caught up in addictions while seeking pleasure, wanting to feel good about ourselves, and the need to throw off the stress, negativity and fear that we continue to create for ourselves here on earth.

Jay says that "the basis for the development of an addiction begins with a thought process that is based on "not feeling safe." This creates actions to do whatever it takes to make you feel safe. This can be picking up a drink, swallowing a pill or ingesting a drug, eating more or less food, or tapping the door three times before you open or close it, or any similar compulsive behavior habit.

This fear of not feeling safe, or loved or good enough or other negative thoughts pushes us to take an action that makes us feel more connected to our higher power where there is nothing but unconditional love, and leads the way to escape from so many negative energies that exist on the earth plane. The catch is that what we may want to escape from can have been created many lifetimes ago yet still exists within us today due to cellular and DNA memory, even genetics that we have carried forward into this lifetime..

And Jay also says that "addiction is a chain of choices." Can you break that chain? Of course you can, though it may not be easy. It is up to you.

Where there is love, there is healing.

CHAPTER I

A GLIMPSE OF JAY

"Just remember that if anything happens to me, I have lived a good life." Upon hearing these words, you may react like I did when my son said this to me several times throughout his teen and later years. You may wonder how a handsome, bright, charming yet addicted person who is so involved with drugs and alcohol and basically a pawn to them means when he says this. He looked at my surprised expression and said, "I mean it." and went on to describe all the ways he had already experienced and enjoyed life.

Meanwhile, I was thinking about how much I wished I could wave a magic wand and begin life again with this child of mine. Would there be something I could do that would change his choices and his pathway in life? Or mine? What mother or father is happy for their son or daughter to experience the kind of life that addiction brings about? What loving parent has not already tried to barter with the Universe to have their child cleared of addictions, even willing to trade places with their child?

How did this even come about?

My son, Jay, was born on a glorious day on May 5, 1969 at 7:18 p.m. He came in with a smile and a glint in his eye. He was always very active and probably could have used Nike sneakers from birth. He loved life and threw himself into it in all ways, some of which turned out not so good. As a tot, he loved adventures from playing in the dirt to splashing in puddles always believing they had been created just for him. From a very early age, Jay seemed to never let anything stop him from enjoying life and having a good time. If you were feeling down, all you had to do was look at his face that bore a grin and you could feel his joy.

At two, he had his stomach pumped several times for drinking forbidden medicine; at three, he was pretending to be superman jumping from the window at Pre-School; at four, he was bringing home dead animals so they wouldn't be lonely. At five, he was diagnosed with a deficiency of the Factor 8 clotting factor, something I carried via my father who had the same condition. It was then that he was bitten by a neighbor's horse and nearly died. At six, his teacher sent home a note suggesting I give him coffee or tea in the morning to keep him calm during school. At seven, he went to a therapist to find out what was going on with him with no results. At eight, Jay's father and I were divorced and life became even more upside down. It had been an abusive marriage and unhappiness flowed down to the children who couldn't understand the behavior, and Jay never had the contact, love and support of his father. At ten, he was smoking cigarettes behind the garage with some of his buddies who had snitched cigarettes from their parents and lied about it. He didn't seem to recognize consequences and would take on a dare without blinking an eye. He loved a challenge, and became a great defender of his friends when they needed his support.

He was always active during the day with a tremendous amount of energy spent in many different ways. Often, at night when he was sleeping, it would become so quiet that many times I would peek into his room just to make sure he was breathing!

He was excellent in sports and when he began to excel in them, he would step away not liking the pressure of continually doing well. He was bored in school, rarely studied, but when pressed to take a test or do a report he would often end up with high grades. He had a photographic memory but was not interested in schooling. Even his therapists were at a loss. Addiction was never brought up as there was no real thinking back then that children could be addicts. All of his negative behavior was something that we all hoped and wished that he would grow out of.

Jay could be delightful for he was a handsome boy who drew people to him. He was sensitive and intuitive even at an early age and could easily recognize if someone was telling the truth or hiding something from him, often walking away from them if he sensed a falseness. He seemed to have a sixth sense about what others expected of him, especially the therapists, and could court them with the answers they wanted to hear. And the therapists seemed to love him and his keen sense of humor – again with no specific diagnosis.

At times, I would be at my wit's end not knowing what to do. There was no internet then, and not much help out there until his later teens when at the age of 18 he went into his first rehab. Throughout his life, he would go into rehab and be able to do well for a length of time and then fall back into his addictions.

During life, Jay enjoyed many different aspects of living. Although he was not a singer or musician, he loved music for it always seemed to soothe his soul. He adored movies and could recite scenes, who played in what role, and could go beyond what had been shown to reach a deeper meaning. He became an excellent cook easily whipping up a tasty meal for family and friends becoming known for his homemade spaghetti sauce and grilling steaks tips, among other things. Children and dogs loved him and the joy of his life was his own son, born nearly three years before his death.

Jay and I had a bond from the beginning, for he was the child that I supposedly wouldn't be able to carry to term due to some issues from previous pregnancies. There was never any doubt that I loved him and that he loved me. That was never a question, although we certainly did not always see eye-to-eye on some of his choices. We provided a safe place for each other to discuss whatever it is we wanted to talk about and we did so often discussing things usually shared between close friends. He would often call me his best friend, and I, him. At times, we discussed spiritual beliefs such as the afterlife, astrology, Karma, how the brain worked, quantum physics, how we fit into life and much more. We both were fascinated by it all!

There is an expression that "what you live, you have created." Many discussions took place around this topic and the importance of who and what you surround yourself with that lends itself to choices and what to do with what you have already created … as an addict, you tend to do some things that you regret later. Jay struggled with that because of remorse. He was like many addicts who can be very tender-hearted, kind and loving who cannot stand some of his actions and choices. So they hop onto the merry-go-round of addiction trying to escape their actions.

All I can say is that it couldn't have been easy to be Jay in this lifetime for so many unpleasant as well as better things and even good things happened to him that it must have been like living nine lives! All I know for sure is that I am very grateful to have had him as my son for many reasons, but the most giving one is what he has taught and remains teaching me each day

Jay's gift to us all is what he shares with us: **We don't die!** He teaches us so much more as we will learn when reading this book. Most of all, he shows us what addiction is and how we can live without addiction NOW.

Where there is love, there is healing.

Chapter 2

What Would Have Made a Difference?

As a frantic parent of an addict who had longed for her child to make different choices, I was haunted by the question, what would have made a difference? Could there have been a different ending? I listed all the "if onlys" blaming myself, the world, God, and everyone else. Then, I would sit quietly, and allow peace to overcome me as I realized I knew better than to get stuck in the whirl wind of addictive thoughts. I didn't really understand how I was able to get into that state of mind - I was just grateful to be there.

Jay's message was always <u>loud and clear</u>: We continue to learn and grow, and we on "the other side" are always with you, helping where we can.

Yet, when Cheryl and I first started our sessions with Jay and the "Others," I still found myself very much like the worried parent wondering if things had been different in our family, would the outcome have been different. So I asked him:

If you had a set of parents with all the love that you needed and you were accepted, would you have been addicted?

He's smiling. He said that I did have all the love I needed and I was accepted so that is a moot point.

*We are going to go beyond into society though. I am going back into some roots of society. I knew that I was loved and accepted but I couldn't FEEL it. But, he says, that is something within **him**.*

And he is going back to society talking about the energy that is prevalent in our society here in the United States right now. He says that energy is where we are so focused on doing, doing, doing and making that the "all-important" that we have forgotten about being. So he is one of those kids who got trapped in not remembering how to be and even though he had all the encouragement to be, it was still about the feeling of being lost from spirit. Losing the connection that is the spirit; that is the hope; that is the love; is addictive itself. The drugs were needed to bring the feeling that should have been felt as spirit.

So many are not focusing on the HEART of spirit, or being spirit, or feeling as the soul, and they look for substitutions. The drugs are the substitutions.

Now you have mentioned in the book "less than" – feeling less than – that is what I am talking about with the doing instead of the being. Whatever you do decides who you are in the eyes of most of society right now and that is a heck of a lot of pressure for a kid. As a kid, you want to have authority, and you feel you should have it, but you really don't. You don't know enough to do what you need to do with your life. The drugs make you feel more than adequate.

So what the drugs do is make you feel as though you can measure up to society while at the same time they give you some of the same kind of feelings that you have when you are connected to soul and connected to spirit. So it is a double whammy.

Jay says that one of the problems is that connecting with spirit takes time and effort. The drugs – you just take a pill. So in our society we have everything instant gratification - right now. So kids growing up now, you have to do it fast, you have to do it immediately, so just pop a pill – it's so much easier.

What would have made a difference for you?

*For me to have been able to **feel** the love I received; for me to be able to look at this measuring stick that we have for everyone that what you do counts not who you are and to be able to know that is false.*

Is there anything else that would have made a difference?

I had a choice this lifetime. What would have made the difference? There are a lot of things that would have made a difference. If I had been able to open my eyes enough to see beyond my helplessness, it would have made a difference. If I had been able to feel the love that was coming from you, from my friends in the physical, from spirit, it would have made a difference. If I had said no the first time, it would have made a difference. If I had changed friends, it would have made a difference.

There are a thousand things that could have made a difference, but it comes down to the final choice; we look at where we are from the soul level and we say I have a 20% chance of coming out of this, I have a 50% chance of hurting someone by doing this. We look at all the possibilities and all the probabilities and we decide whether or not it is to the highest good of self to continue. And other people's well-being has to be brought into this.

For example, unknowingly, when I was checking on myself saying this is where I stand, I knew that the addiction was going to get much, much, worse. I knew that I was going to continue to go downhill because I didn't feel I had the strength to fight it and, frankly, I didn't want to spend the rest of my life fighting an addiction, and I didn't see any way around it. But I could also see what I would be doing to you. Even though you say nothing could be worse than not having you that is not true. I also saw what I would be doing to a young lady that I cared about very much, and I realized that this could be turned into a win by sending a message through you.

Now, you and I had made the agreement prior to my coming in as your son that if this was the outcome, we would do this work together We both prayed for the outcome of beating the addiction and do the work that way in the physical, but it wasn't moving in that direction. So we decided to do it Plan B.

You know, Mom, if I had been able to feel how much you loved me, it would have made all the difference in the world. I can see it now; I can feel it now. But it was something inside ME that wouldn't receive it as a healing balm.

WHY DID YOU CHOOSE THE FATHER YOU DID?

That goes into the obsessive compulsive behaviors. It brought up that I am not safe. He came in deliberately with his father to bring up, "I am not safe," to bring it to the surface to clear it. You were his chance to clear it. He's got the two opposites for parents. He also wanted to work on the acceptance of "self regardless of how someone else feels about you." He says that he did get some work done on that. So that was very important. So in some sense, his father was a very important teacher. Jay says that his father was absolutely perfect for making him feel he was never safe. And that is what he was trying to bring to surface. That is what he was trying to wrestle with. So it was a perfect choice in that sense.

Jay says. "I chose the right guy."

"Well, *I* certainly didn't choose the right guy."

Yes, you did because of what you and Jay are working out and because of the issues you brought in. Look at how much stronger and wiser you are because of Jay's father.

"That's true. I guess I will have to get to the point of thanking him."

Jay is laughing, "I want to see that. That is one of the things you need to work on before you leave, Mom."

Jay says if you can't love this person, can you love him through me? He says you are reaching the point with your ex-husband of truly being able to give up any kind of having to be the judge.

It is interesting because Jay says this last part is the hardest because it is about your kids – you screwed up my kids' lives. You were not nice to them and you were not loving to them. The challenge is to see them as the good souls that they are instead of your children.

Jay says, "You'll do it."

JAY, WHAT ARE YOU WORKING ON?

I am working with Masters in the 7th dimension as part of my expansion of consciousness to learn and grow as much as I can before I take embodiment again. And just so you know, on a scale of one to ten, when I left I was not a 10. I was an 8. A 10 is someone who is completely addicted, never sees daylight, and is angry or severely depressed and non-functional. I was able to fake it sometimes and I was able to feel good sometimes, thanks in large part to you. So I crossed over as an 8 rather than a 10.

Now the work that I am doing in the 5th dimension, a lot of it has been healing me of ties that were created of the physical body while I was there. Now I am working on the specific vibrational frequencies and addictions as a part of preparing myself for re-embodiment because I am still very, very hopeful that I will be able to conclude the addiction pattern in the earth plane. The more that I can assist and can come to an understanding on this side, the less the pressure on me so that I can cross over as an 8. But, depending on the work I do on this side, how long I do it, and the intensity, I can come back into my next lifetime as a 6 or 7.

SO YOU STILL COME IN WITH ADDICTION? BECAUSE IT TAKES LIFETIMES — IS THAT WHAT YOU ARE SAYING?

I could. I actually could. If I can bring it down to a 6 or 7, I could end my addiction in my next lifetime. It isn't guaranteed because it is still a 6 or 7, but it is much, much more likely than the chunk that I bit off this lifetime.

DO YOU THINK THAT YOUR PARENTS AND FAMILY MEMBERS THIS LIFETIME WERE A DETERRENT?

Actually, the family members are the reason I crossed over as an 8 instead of a 10. Yes, some of them were problematic. Dad was problematic, etc. However, the fact that I always had a central source of support from my family, two members in particular, you being the primary, made a huge difference. As an addict, I stayed longer that I have before, believe it or not, the crossover was not in complete rage, and it wasn't violent in the sense of trying to lash out at someone or hating myself or anything of that nature. It was more of a corner and not knowing what to do, and that is a huge difference. One of the reasons I chose the family was that I bit off more than I could chew. I looked at it and said "Oh no, I want it this strong."

He is rolling his eyes at himself.

JAY, WHAT ARE YOU DOING ON OTHER SIDE?

Remember the movie Limitless? He says, only it's really, really, different from that movie. In that movie the guy did for doing, processing, etc. It isn't as if there is a frantic need to do here. There is a joy in doing as a service. There is so much to learn, so much to see, so much! He says, imagine this as a huge universe with thousands of classes to choose from and you want to take every single one of them, times it by 100,000, and I want to take every single one of them.

JAY, DO YOU SEE ANYONE ELSE — ANYONE IN THE FAMILY? MY MOTHER AND FATHER?

Sometimes. We are not studying exactly the same thing but we often meet, sometimes in a family gathering or picnic; sometimes we cross paths in the library; sometimes we just get together to say hi, talk about what is going on, and check on you.

He's a part of the family group. He sees his uncle and is working with him in one of the groups. Jay is working in 5 or 6 different groups.

Let me explain a little bit how the family units work here. Here on earth, we have separation with one family here, another family there, etc. On this side, we think of it as yes, we are one huge family, but certain members of the family have much more interaction with each other than other members of the family.

So you would look at it as my family is 1,000 souls (he is just picking numbers out of the air for us) and I work very closely with 300 of them. We can live together; we can manifest houses; we can sleep or don't sleep; whatever we want to do. Relationships with each other means if we want to have a family reunion type of gathering, we can! The reunions are interesting because it is not just members of the family this lifetime, but is with members from the lifetime of the 18th century, the 14th century from all over the map and earth. He says to expand, expand; we are part of the universe up here.

He says that it is the same way with the groups who work together. He's talking about this group of say 1,000 where there are 5 or 6 different themes they share. They each have a certain level of interest in a theme that they are assisting with – whether they are helping with the dimensions that are lost or the ones going to a new level – whatever, it is doesn't matter. He says that some of that group will be absolutely fascinated by faction one of it so we will work intensely on faction one whereas we will be a sort of poor thrill group for faction 4. Now, take every single individual in that group with their varying likes and dislikes and apply it to every faction of what they want done.

SO WHAT ARE THE DIFFERENT THEMES?

He says that in this case, the one he is really interested in as far as the Japan thing is when he was talking about mass consciousness thoughts being released to be cleared. It literally opened fissures of ancient energy coming up to be cleared. He says that relates directly to addictions. Our thought patterns are beliefs that we accept from someone else without even knowing that we accepted it is an addiction. It is such a close addiction, we don't even know it.

Example: someone who is told he is fat as a child. It is an addiction because it is now a belief and they are willing to own it as a belief. They feel so stuck with it they can't get rid of it – that is an addict. Any kind of addiction modifies the thought feeling behavior. In other words, the belief I am fat completely modifies that individual's thoughts, feelings, and behavior. It is the emotion that takes over the behavior. He says that the problem is they have been in it since day 1 so they don't even realize what is going on.

What is that step that triggers that they don't have to be that addict?

He says the ultimate thing that HAS to happen is that they HAVE to have an idea – a moment in faith, that their lives could be better and they are stronger than they realize.

Is it will?

Will is based on logical facts. You need to go to level of faith. We are going to go down into the emotional, we are going to have that spark of feeling that we are strong and able even if it is for just a split second. Then, if we can hang onto that and recreate that anytime with anybody's help, then we have a ladder to crawl on, something that makes us feel better than the addiction does - something to escape TO instead of using the addiction to escape FROM.

It sounds like they develop their own high?

It comes down to the point that they have to see themselves as what and who they really are or at least know that it is possible. He says that anyone who is caught in addiction believes that he cannot do or be without whatever he is addicted to. Therefore, he is weak in the sense that something else has to empower him. He can have that flash of empowerment in himself by knowing himself as he is, and not knowing himself as an addict or whatever he has taken on to own. Empowerment is just a flash of knowing yourself.

THANK YOU. LOVE YOU.

Love you, too.

Where there is love, there is healing.

CHAPTER 3

HOW DID IT ALL BEGIN?

I was beginning to understand. I wanted to know more. I had a driving need for Jay to share with us not only addiction in general, but more about his own addictions. When did they start? Was I involved? Was I at fault?

I was curious to know how he reviewed things, particularly in light of it now being in "hindsight," if you will, and his ability to look at addiction without the veil between dimensions. What is addiction, really?

The more that I listened to what the whole group said and re-read what I had transcribed, the more I found myself mesmerized in what Jay was sharing, especially about himself. And the gift of it all was that I was better able to accept more of who I am as a spirit in human form with all the flaws of living in this heavy third dimension. Hopefully, you will, too.

So I asked:

HOW DO YOU EXPLAIN ADDICTION?

*Addictions are intense, compacted, and becoming extreme to light or darkness. They have become a Prime Threat going to one extreme or another. **Addiction is about unawareness** – unawareness that every second we are alive, we are choosing consciously or unconsciously - an unawareness that we have power always every second to choose differently. Addiction is about getting stuck – think of a hamster on a wheel going around and around.*

All it takes is just one split second of awareness to come out of addiction. The way we look at it now is we think of it as being 20 years of Alcoholic Anonymous. Because of the intensity of addiction and our choices, we have outgrown that aspect of it. If we can only realize that it is not a great big giant effort that we are going to have to stay sober and fight it every second of our life for the rest of our lives.

*Who is going to want to face that? What we are finally beginning to understand is that it is a split second choice here, a split second of awareness there ... it's being nice to ourselves. It is shifting that split second at a time where we lighten up. We no longer look at it as an addiction; we look at it as **a chain of choices.** Addiction means that we are stuck, that we have to fight and struggle, chain of choices means we choose differently.*

The willingness to look at that power to choose as glory and fun and a thrilling exciting ride instead of a heavy responsibility and duty.

WERE YOU BORN ADDICTED?

Yes, I was born addicted. When I came into this lifetime, I asked that the cellular memory of addiction be strong enough to be in my face. I over-estimated my ability. I was warned to make it less, but I really, really wanted to change it in this lifetime so I bit off more than I could chew.

Addiction can be carried through family trees – genetics. I came in with an addictive belief system. I am addicted to the thought that I am not enough without outside influences.

Knowing that Jay had been born addicted, I wanted to understand how that can be. I wanted to know when his addictions began. I asked him if he would share some lives regarding DNA, cellular memory, and more so that I could have a better grasp of how everything works. I was very surprised at what he told us and how his explanation covered so much, yet was so simple. The more I read and re-read what he said it makes so much sense to me to see where we are today with so many problems that could easily be changed with inward being and thinking connecting us to source– always with love, especially with love and acceptance of self.

Jay continually reminds us: "Learn to love and all addiction will cease." He also says that "Anything that is held from love cannot be healed."

Here is what Jay shared with us about his own addictions:

THE BEGINNING OF ADDICTIONS RE: DNA

"Let's go clear back to when we first started taking form in the physical world before what we think of as a dense body. He is showing a progression. Imagine he is coming down as the soul taking no body yet at all with a whole bunch of others like a sea of people coming down with some of the masters and a whole group of teachers. And the planet is ready. There have already been a few brave pioneer souls who have stepped into it but not very many at all, just the higher level ones have so far. There is a whole sea of people who have asked to be able to evolve in this dimension.

He said that at that time it wasn't the school of hard knocks that it is now. It was a beautiful planet; it was just a different kind of dimension so we could enjoy different kinds of experiences, but everyone who came there was still very, very connected with the source. We all knew who and what we were and were just experiencing it in another dimension.

It looks like a large orientation group. We were shown around the planet like a tour of a college campus. We were all in awe of just how beautiful this planet was and how unique it was because even then it was unlike anything else anywhere in the dimensions. There was such a rich texture of being able to touch. Even in the spirit body we could touch because the plants were three dimensional, the trees, the animals - it was just fascinating! We all were very excited about coming here.

They talked to us about the fact that when we came here, we would still know who we are, but because it was such a very unique experience, we needed to be careful not to shift our focus. Look at it like children. You want them to play with safe toys and with one that stretches them a bit every now and then. It is a good idea, but you don't want them to do it all the time.

For example, you have a child and you want that child to play with Legos most of the time, but he is older now and developing motor skills so you want him to ride his bike, too. We were told that the temptation would be to become completely immersed in the joys of the sensations which weren't called physical sensations at the time, rather were called earth plane sensations. Jay says that the planet was not called earth at that time. That the name earth came quite a bit later.

WHAT WAS IT CALLED?

One of the more recent in the ancient history was called terra. He said that at one point it was called the orb of vision - that was when it was in the developing stages – and they just called it the orb. He is kind of chuckling. He says it's kind of like when scientists attach names to their experiments - sometimes it makes sense and sometimes it doesn't. But it is fascinating that they would call it the orb of vision when it is 3D and we think of it as just the opposite - flat.

He says, "Well, that is because it didn't go as planned, did it?"

He is in a huge sea of people in the orientation group with a bunch of masters, higher guides and teachers and talking about what is going on and everyone is "oohing" and "aahing" and it looks much like a cub scout group at a wild life preserve, and most are very, very excited. He said that between one fourth and one third decided not to come here because when the teachers were talking about the possibility of becoming fascinated by these experiences outside of self, they didn't feel they were strong enough to resist it and they weren't going to risk it.

WHERE WERE THEY COMING FROM?

He says all over the universe. He says there are individuals from every

CHAPTER 3 - HOW DID IT ALL BEGIN?

planet and a lot of different dimensions. The call went out for anyone who is interested in evolving in a different way. So in orientation they are looking at the orb as pristine, absolutely clean and clear of what we call germs, bacteria, mosquitoes and predators. It is the paradise the bible talks about. He says that the earth plane was the Garden of Eden - the entire planet - not just a physical location.

He says that a bunch of them decided to move ahead. There are a lot of layers of groups, but he is narrowing it down to five main groups going in at different times. The most highly advanced are going in first. They are there over a 1,000 years before the next group goes in. Everything is running fine. The more highly evolved group has informed everyone that, yeah, it would be really easy to slip into absolute fascination like an obsession, but it is a wonderful way to learn and grow and the experiences are truly unique.

He is in the 3rd wave, and when the 2nd wave comes in, everything is going okay. It's a little bit tougher because there are more people involved, and the more that are involved in an experiment, it is harder to keep the control and maintain that higher level.

When he comes in on the 3rd wave, by that time it still was very, very, beautiful and it was pristine in the sense no predators, no germs, etc. but the shift and the feeling had already started. The shift and the feeling was as if children went to a playground or Disney Land - remember Pinocchio? Children went to a play thing and forgot all about home, and they lived there and that was their only reality. That is what was starting already, just barely, so there was some concern about that. So they were given lots of different orientation classes and a great deal of training with the methods of individualized focus - the centering himself and staying there.

Sometime just as the 4th wave came something happened. There was some sort of shift and rift going on. The shift or the rift was not supposed to happen. It is one of those cosmic things. The 4th wave had already started to come in and it was decided that it was too late to stop it. The shift affected the balance of negative/positive in the earth plane. At that time, all those who were there, it is like they were affected with that.

Those that were very highly evolved just got a tiny bit of that and were able to brush it off. But anyone not highly-evolved, the tainting of the DNA started at that point. And he is showing it as there is some kind of power struggle going on. Like there is this beautiful, pristine planet with its only purpose evolution and loving God and spreading this energy through the universe.

It sounds traumatic, but they are showing that the entities, beings, souls, whatever you want to call them who were existing in the darker planes, got really angry because they were not allowed in. There was not supposed to be a mixing of the energies. It was supposed to be taking those in levels one through five (levels 4 and 5 were what you would think of as just good ordinary people taking the human form and going to the 5th dimension when they cross over; they were decent human beings).

The first level that came in is closer to master level and included some masters just to assist. Imagine if word got out to the wrong people that there was a nirvana waiting …. Imagine in our current day and age, if we had a community where there were no guns, no one was allowed to fight, and they had all kinds of wealth, you know how that would attract the bad guys? Well, word wasn't supposed to get out to that dimension, but somehow it did.

How are you going to stop energy? Energy connects to energy. There was some kind of a power struggle in the non-physical dimension and when that happened, they are literally showing a rift opening up. The rift is affecting everything with the ripple effect. Like the tsunami in Japan. How it hit that one spot, but then the repercussions just kept going and going. It would flood another shore; it would be a hurricane or a tornado over there. This is what happened with the energetic rift, and there was a little bit of an opening in the protective atmosphere around earth.

Did I come in with you, Jay?

He is winking at you. Yes, you came in on the 3rd wave also. The 4th wave came in and at that point, think of that as a rift in the energy grid - he says that's the best way to look at it. It's an energy grid that was disturbed. Once that *energy grid was disturbed, we now knew negative energy. We had it. It was a part of the system; it was an infectious germ that everyone now had to deal with.*

He said they had thought about not letting the 5th wave in and, in fact, they delayed it for thousands of years because of what was going on. But then they decided to let the 5th wave come in because they had worked for the privilege of coming in and helping for all those thousands of years, specifically for that, so they were hoping to create a better balance, but it just keep getting worse and worse.

They are pointing to that story of Adam and Eve in the Garden of Eden. They are saying that the apple represents the negativity going into the emotions (think of the human emotions instead of the emotions of the soul: joy, patience, compassion, etc.).

The emotions of humans are pleasure/pain and any derivative of those two. You and he in that wave were okay for a while, but think of it as a group of 20 people and the infection comes in and everyone is fine taking your medicine, vitamin C, and fighting it. In this case, you all were doing your spiritual work, keeping your proper focus and then one gets just a little bit sick and everyone looks at this as okay, we are going to gather our energy and heal this one.

That one wasn't able to take in that energy because the sickness was actually a shifting to more focus on the negative energy instead of the positive energy. And all it took was just that one little shift. It was 100% positive, then it was 99% positive, then 98% positive. Think of it as this was the first one to slip below 90% positive. That means that the infection has a foothold.

They are working on clearing this, but the problem was that while working on clearing this, that very act of clearing it gave them a feeling of the reality of the negative energy. So it was like a catch 22. By helping this person clear it, they were acknowledging it was a reality, and by acknowledging it as a reality, they helped feed it. So most of the healing they were doing was good, like 90% of it was good, but 10% was shoring up the reality of negative energy ... the illusion that had been created.

SO WAS I IN THAT GROUP OF 20?

No, he is just using that as an example so that we would understand it in earth plane terms. It actually took place on a much, much larger scale. In groups of thousands, 20 would lapse in their vigilance and went into the negativity as a reality (so when you recognize it, you create it). And before, they were able to know it was a reality that did not fit on the earth plane because it was a negative thing that had been created in other dimensions. It was not God created, it was God's creatures created. Ultimately everything is God created.

Imagine that this has just happened and now there is an issue with the DNA and with the earth itself, and as the switch was made, it then became a part of the "human form" because we were still in pretty light bodies at that time. In fact, we were in very light bodies but once that shift started, the bodies started to become denser and denser because our minds were pulled toward the negativity, the fear, and at the same time toward finding something to fix it.

Then finding something to fix it became an outward thing instead of an inward thing and it was kind of the domino effect over hundreds of thousands of years from that. He is saying that it was never considered to just pull people off the planet and give up because life is life, and life continues to grow and expand, etc. All change is possible.

He says there were several points there. Remember Noah and the Ark? That's actually being handed down from a time period where the negativity of the earth plane became so heavy it was bringing everyone and everything down with it and the earth was purged. It's a symbolic representation, of course. They are saying what happened was the purest of the light forms that were the least tainted were pulled off the surface and everyone leaves like a lot of us are leaving now, getting ready for the purge. That's the symbolism of Noah's Ark and the water is spirit. Most of the people there died before the flooding came. He says the floods are very, very real. The story is symbolic, but the cleansing of the earth with water is very real. He says that we have done that dozens of times.

In more modern times have we cleansed the earth with flooding and tsunamis?

That is on a lesser scale, yes. He says that dozens of times we have literally cleansed the earth plane with water and completely changed the land structures and everything. Yes, but things like the tsunami is a smaller version of that and we are hoping will work so we don't have to do the other one again - the same with the earth quakes. He is saying that some of the earthquakes are caused by disruption, and some are deliberately set with the agreement of the souls involved to help release the pressure of the negativity.

He says that, in a nutshell, that is how millions and millions of years progressed until we have the physical bodies we have now and what you might call the DNA of addiction. (Basically, DNA stands for the building structure.)

Adamantine Particles is the term currently being used for the energy substance that is the essence of all creation everywhere and everything that is uncreated. It is the building block that contains all potential. We are saying DNA because we are talking about the physical human form of addictions and that sort of thing. So we are going to use DNA, but the fact is that it was the adamantine particles themselves, the ones that had already been shifted to something else here on the earth plane that became infected. It's not the original adamantine particles, they are always pure, but it is all the stuff we were using to create, kind of like you have a vat of liquid that you are going to create with and you put in one drop of poison. The whole vat is affected that way.

Now he says that tying that into the story he just told us, the addiction started with the fascination with the power of fighting off the negativity, not realizing that we were helping to build it because it gave us something to flex our muscles against. He says that it went from obsession to fascination, with the being able to overpower negativity to the fascination of how else to do it. We began to look at plants, animals, the air and causes outside the creator, outside of self. He says that at that point, we were caught. So again, it is when you focus and look outward instead of inward that you have problems.

And taking it a step further, it is outward instead of inward based in fear instead of love. Take a look at Mother Teresa. She is always focused inward living the energy of love, but is also outwardly focused because she stays strong in faith. She never lets the negativity touch the hem of her garment. And when we focused outward, it wasn't us focusing our inner strength outward; it was us focusing on the negativity of the outward. Not in the sense of "It's scary, scary," but in the sense of "Oh, look at that!" It was that we went from inner to outer. He says that has been the key problem forever.

Jay's Early Lifetimes Demonstrating DNA

He says that now that he has laid the ground work, if you would like to, he can go through some personal lives.

1. *So he is going to go to a lifetime when it still wasn't very dense. You guys had lost the ability to completely transport yourselves in spirit, body, and thinking – wherever you need to be or whoever you need to be, etc. In this lifetime, he says that you had already lost all that except for a few masters that were still there -there were about a dozen of them still holding the planet from the surface of the planet. Of course, there were thousands and millions of them in the non-physical.*

Now in that lifetime - he is showing me a picture of explorers like the famous guides like Lewis & Clark, Livingston and all those people. You and he were in a massive group of people who were absolutely fascinated by the textures, sights, sounds and touch of the earth plane. He says that you hadn't moved into taste yet. You didn't need it. You were absolutely fascinated by those senses because at that time, there was nothing available anywhere else in the universe. And you guys used to go out on expeditions, and it was still a light enough body that you could cover an awful lot of ground and you could go under the water. He says that your favorite was actually going under the water because you loved the colors under there. That in itself became an addiction for both of us.

For him, it was the addiction to the excitement of discovery. And we might think of that as a positive addiction, but he says that an addiction is an addiction. Too much of a good thing is too much. And it assisted in pulling to the outward focus. The fascination with those senses was like a little kid playing a video game instead of eating something healthy. He says that in that lifetime you could consider that addiction as a healthy one except before that, you guys had been mostly inner processing, still very connected, still very aware of who you are.

It wasn't as easy as it used to be, but you were almost completely in the knowing that threw you out of it. **It's the addiction of adventure, the addiction of new highs.** He says that it is the newness. We never knew what we were going to find and where we were going to find it. And, of course, you get to report it back to all your friends and they come to look at it and it just becomes a huge party. It was feeding the emotions that you didn't even know you had. That was part of creating the human emotions of the pleasure/pain cycle because in that process you began to feel the first inklings of disappointment when you didn't find anything new or exciting.

He says that **addiction creates the absolute guarantee of disappointment sooner or later.** That fits with what they say about attachment. **Addiction is an attachment to the feeling you get from a result** – the result of finding something new and exciting. Attachment like that is an automatic guarantee of disappointment. He says that is what they are really talking about when they say to detach – learn not to become attached to anything. **The "desireless desire."**

2. This next lifetime is the perfect example of going into the desire. He says that this is actually a collage of many lifetimes. He is simplifying it or otherwise we would be talking about a lot of different lifetimes. He says that it was important to lay the basics of that first lifetime when you and he were both involved in that. He said that you didn't get quite as addicted as he did. You enjoyed it, but you were still in a space where you enjoyed a natural communing – a crystal time – you look like a crystal, this wonderful beautiful etched energy and you really loved it.

He says that he did too, but this was a new exciting toy for him.

We are all in pretty dense physical bodies, not like we are now, but very close. In this lifetime, I learned that someone could take away what I need. So take the negativity, the addiction, the searching for the high of finding something new and exciting. In this lifetime, I discovered the high of someone looking at me as if I am god. I had no idea that I had missed that. I had no idea that I wasn't thinking of myself as one with the creator anymore. He says that he got into the addiction so heavily that he didn't know he was addicted. It wasn't god in the sense that he was the God of all creation, it was god in the sense of "you are my hero." It was a very human thing, but it was the closest thing he had felt in that in a very, very, long time.

Remember the Pinocchio story? He says that he had fallen into being there to where he forgot he had ever known he was one with God. It didn't exist. So when this other human form came in and said, "Oh my gosh! You are so wonderful! You are so fabulous, etc."

That was the first time he had felt that kind of charge in many, many centuries. That is when he became addicted to that feed because he wasn't getting that energy feed from anywhere else. He was in male form that lifetime and it was a female form that gave him that feed. He didn't know that part of what was happening is that they recognized each other. They were part of the same group – part of that third wave that came in. She recognized him; he didn't, but she didn't know why she was recognizing him. She just knew that there was an immediate attachment to the fact that he was wonderful and life would be good with him. She didn't realize that she was picking up on who they used to be.

SO FOR ALL THOSE CENTURIES YOU WERE ALWAYS LOOKING FOR MORE?

Exactly.

For a long time he was looking for the excitement of discovery of playing on the earth plane and that after how many centuries it was this came up, a brand new addiction a thousand times more fierce than the other – a thousand times headier. So that's when he started the addiction of the **needing someone to love him in the human form.** *At that time, most of us were too – most of us had lost ourselves and were just coming into the discovery of getting that charge from other human beings. He says that it had only been going on for a couple thousand years, which to them on the other side is like a drop of water in the ocean. He says that you have to remember, too, that time was different on the earth plane back then. What we think of a year here could have taken place a thousand years there.*

But at this phase, the linear time was also slowing way down. We had created that as well with the separation. He says that it didn't go well because, of course, if you don't know your "God-self," you cannot be the god that someone else thinks they need you to be. So that is when he learned to keep looking for that love from the opposite sex.

He says that the next lifetime he came in as a female instead of a male because he was hoping to be able to balance out that need of love from the opposite sex. He is rolling his eyes saying that didn't work either. So that was the addiction of getting that love charge from someone else. Now put together the fact that I had an addiction for adventure, basically, exploration and finding new and exciting new things. Then I had an addiction for getting a charge of someone loving me, which is up the ladder from the original addiction. **Now I can't get the feed I need from someone loving me because it doesn't work if you don't love yourself.**

3. *Now we go into another lifetime where there is a substance that can make you remember that you are one. It's not the same thing, but he is likening it to that liquid that the ancient tribe used to put you into a vision state. He says think of it as a chance to experience that kind of drug when you are so down he has worked himself into a state of desperation and he is pretty miserable by this lifetime. And someone says that if you take this, all your troubles disappear and it's natural, we make it out of plants and it makes you feel good so it is like medicine. It's a*

*hallucinogen. He says that was the **addiction to chemical substances** right there and he says that we have to be careful how we call it an addiction to chemical substance because **it is not really an addiction to chemical substance, it really is an addiction to the results**.*

*Yes, the body can create an addiction because of the chemical changes that are created or bio-chemical changes, but he says the truth of the matter is it's the **feeling** state that the drug takes you into that you are addicted to. It's like chocolate, you don't want the result to be pounds on your hips; you want the result to be feeling good. He had gone many, many thousands of years not knowing himself as God, not even knowing God for that matter, even knowing God outside of self. And here he was suddenly one with everything and all powerful. And he says that at that point he began an addictive search for that feeling outside of self instead of inside self because in his mind it came from that liquid.*

HAVE YOU LEARNED TO LOVE YOURSELF?

*Much more than before, yes. However, he had not in that lifetime, of course, for he had no idea. He was still chasing around. He says I didn't know God from Sikkim. Since then, there have been an awful lot of hard knocks and he has learned to love himself and laugh at who he used to be. He says that is very important. **The more we get down on ourselves, the more we are vulnerable to the lower vibrations, the more the addiction holds us captive.** So the more that we can learn to love ourselves, to give ourselves a break and even laugh with ourselves over what we have done, the more that we break free from the addiction.*

IS THERE ANOTHER LIFETIME TO RELATE?

He says no, those three will represent the major stages. He says isn't it ironic that in our original state our experiences were bliss then we became addicted to experiences outside of self because we wanted to feel bliss and because we wanted to feel excitement and all that good stuff? He's just kind of chuckling. We get ourselves into a state of "it's never enough." And it is't because we are looking outside of self instead of inside self.

BEFORE WE END, CAN YOU EXPLAIN DNA IN GREATER DETAIL?

When you are looking at DNA, think of it as a complete and complex system, much more complex than, for example, the intricate clockwork in that every single piece is needed for the system to function properly. If you affect one piece, if you take it out, if you misshape it, if anything is wrong with one piece of it, the entire system has to either adjust to make up for the difference in that piece which will, of course, create a dependency on a different way of moving, a different way of being. If anything is changed in that system, the entire system becomes dependent on a new source of being.

So let's look at it from the human standpoint where you have trillions upon trillions of aspects coming together to create what we think of as human form and all of the bodies that operate in synchronicity with the human form. When you are in the physical body itself, every gland, every organ, every little bitty piece, even those you haven't discovered yet, plays a role in the balance of helping to keep the body healthy. If you interfere with any of that, you have messed with the entire system that now has to adjust accordingly.

A simple way of looking at it is if you have a vertebra out of place in the spine, all muscles and tendons and what they are hooked to has to adjust to compensate. So let's say, for example, you take a hit off a marijuana joint, and when you take that hit you are now completely altering chemicals and in this sense they are being altered in a negative way. They are either being subdued or are being agitated. They need that balance just like a pendulum clock needs that balance for the pendulum to swing.

Each time you put anything negative into the body, whether it is food, liquid, thought, emotion or some substance of abuse, you are knocking that clock off balance. The pendulum now has to adjust in order to work at all and is not going to keep the perfect time it kept before.

The more you do this to the body, the more it becomes accustomed to the new way of being. So once again, back to the drugs. Once you take that hit of the joint, the body is now taking it in and getting the release of all these great feeling chemicals where we relax. What is happening is those parts of the brain that are specifically made to function precisely are being told to be quiet. They are being calmed down, numbed if you will, and each time you do that, the body has to make an adjustment to be able to survive, to be able to move, and have its being within that space you have created. The more you do that, the more the body looks at that as the normal space and previously balanced and healthy state as the abnormal state. So the more you do it, the more the body will seek it because it is saying: Oh, that's where I am supposed to be - the mind, emotions - the same way.

So each time you do this, there is a greater pull to do it again. Now, if you take one hit and you never take another one, no harm done. The problem is that feel good stuff that we get from it. There is a memory tied into every aspect of the human existence, tied into the judgment of pleasure and pain. It's judged as pleasurable; it's judged as painful.

If you take a hit of a marijuana joint, you are going into a state of relaxation that feels very pleasurable for most people. There is a memory of pleasure vs. the stress of living, so there's always a thought in the back of the mind that says, well, if things get too bad, I can always do that again. So you have two things going at the same time. You have the drive toward pleasure which is the basic survival instinct, and you have the system trying to figure out what normal is, what healthy or homeostatic (equilibrium) is. That is on the DNA level.

Also on the DNA level, we have to look at the influence of past lives. We are everything we have ever been — we are that accumulative energy. Even though we look at ourselves as the human form — the human form is the microcosmic condensation of energetic particles that represent where we are in our evolvement. So anything that we have done in the past comes forward with us. Now sometimes we will bring certain aspects very strongly and other aspects we will wait and deal with another lifetime. But when you are dealing with issues of addiction, it affects all areas of the being. You said at one time it is not so much that I am addicted to a specific subject, but that I am an addict.

He is going into the branch of life that goes into the past lives. Think of it as every child is affected by DNA of their parents. Every child is also affected by the DNA of every parent it has ever had, every child it has ever had, every lifetime to one degree or another. So if we look at that we come to realize what a truly tangled web it is.

IS CELLULAR MEMORY DIFFERENT FROM DNA?

The way it is being defined right now is cells are those aspects of the human body that construct the human body. The other is being defined as what is called the adamantine particles, which are pure creation energy. That is the way people are differentiating it right now.

IS CELLULAR MEMORY SOUL MEMORY?

For all intents and purposes, yes. It is the energetic memory of everything you have ever been. It is never lost. It can change but it never dies; it is never lost. And there are levers you can use for the cellular memory. For example, each lifetime that you go into you are working on a specific theme and you will look at your cellular memory and say, I want this part of cellular memory to be very, very, strong, and I would like this other part to be somewhat muted. It's like remembering on a conscious level and, in a way, this part of my cellular memory will come up to be addressed in this lifetime more obviously.

SO WHEN THEY ARE TALKING ABOUT CELLULAR MEMORY, THEY ARE REALLY TALKING ABOUT ENERGY MEMORY?

Exactly. Cells are pure energy or rather just energy because sometimes they are pure and sometimes they are tainted. But pure energy in the sense that nothing else is involved and is energy of the whole being from the beginning to having no end.

IS YOUR HIGHER SELF YOUR SOUL SELF?

Yes.

IS YOUR HIGHER POWER GOD OR IS IT YOUR SOUL SELF?

It depends upon who you are talking to because we are using different labels for the same thing. You can boil it down to your higher self is that aspect that has never lost connection with God so you might call it your God self. Some people will look at it and say it is one and the same thing and others will say no they are two distinctly different things but what you are talking about is gradation of connection.

I CALL THE HIGHER SELF MY "INNER KNOWINGS," WHICH IS THAT ASPECT OF GOD, THAT PART OF SELF THAT IS STILL PART OF GOD AND THAT IS WHAT COMES THROUGH.

We say higher self, but we can really call it God. We could call it God self if we wanted to, but as we introduce this information, we try to be careful to do it in steps where it is more palatable. Many people can hear higher power but if you say it's you as God, they have trouble with that. You might say the higher self is the "I AM." Now some people will also label it as the soul is that part of the adamantine factor of the individual that has gotten tied up somewhat in the third dimension.

We looked at Jay's developing behaviors from **an addiction of highs and new adventures to an addiction to desire to an addiction to chemicals**.

I asked Jay if next time he would share some other of his lifetimes that would simply show us different *types* of addiction, which he has laid out for us in the next chapter.

THANK YOU. LOVE YOU.

Love you, too.

Where there is love, there is healing.

Chapter 4

Can You Share Different Lifetimes of Addictions?

After hearing what Jay was sharing, and knowing that he had opened the door on my own addictions from a long, long time ago - the addiction to color and texture - I looked around my house and saw many items that confirm that. If I am outside walking, I am always commenting on the color of things because I find Nature's colors soothing. It became very clear to me that, indeed, we do carry forward our addictions. Now I was determined to understand in a clear way how that worked. And I knew that Jay could help me.

So I asked him:

Jay, would you be willing to share some of your lifetimes with us so that we can understand the concept of bringing forth addictions?

He says, that for him, he is going to go way back in time where the addiction actually started as a thought addiction, not a substance one. He is going back at a time when fear became my thought addiction. We are going clear back in time where time is not even recorded. He says that he got into a lifetime where it was constant threat of non-survival. It was REAL constant threat of non-survival; think about fighting animals like the saber tooth cats. They are very mean looking.

He says way back in that time period, he got locked into the fear addiction because it was part of a survival mode. It was one of those things where you had to be constantly looking - you couldn't even sleep without that monitor on — like soldiers.

He says that it was a part of life where he was one of those in the group of people where it was his job to watch out for their well-being. About half the group had that job because they were very good at being alert, watching and all that stuff. He says that he spent that entire lifetime expecting disaster, trauma, blood, the whole nine yards He got locked into it; he didn't let go. Most of that group he was with got locked into it. He then lived a few lifetimes where there was obviously not the immediate threat of survival at all times to try to help calm that down, and he says that it did help lessen it, but it was always in the background.

He says that in those lifetimes, I didn't recognize why I was so anxious all the time and I'd keep looking for the reason. Sometimes, I could find something and think maybe that was the reason, but I never really knew what it was. It never came to a point of awareness. He is showing a tie in as far as emotions and energy.

In that lifetime where we were constantly fighting for survival there was the energy of the fear that says we have to be aware all the time, we have to be careful, we have to have hiding holes, we have to have things planned ahead for disaster, all of this stuff. Think of the emotions and the energies that attach to the threat of survival.

He says we are going to go into addictive behaviors for him again, not addictive in the sense of drugs, but in the sense of obsessive compulsive. We are going to go into the next significant lifetime where it became obsessive compulsive behavior.

In this lifetime, I did not understand where it was coming from and I had that kind of thought mentality that said I have to watch, I have to be very careful to make sure that everything is exactly the way it needs to be to survive — obsessive compulsive behavior. He says that now the emotion of fear of death tied into the first lifetime. *He is now trying to control the emotion of fear of death because he doesn't know what it is, doesn't know where it is coming from. Therefore, he can't take care of it. By making certain that everything is done just so and he has absolute control over every little thing he says drove people crazy in that lifetime!*

He is going to a time period that we would think of it like Victorian England, but a long time before that — it's one of the similar cycles before that — where he locks doors three times: you lock it to make sure it works, you unlock it, you open it to make sure you unlocked it, you lock it. You do that three times. Then you go back and check it three times. He set up all these rituals to make sure everything is safe. No fun at all. He says it actually was worse than the animals trying to kill us. So everything in his life had to have rituals. He is showing himself going to work in something like a bank, looking like the old Victorian banks, and every time he had to touch the door knob just once. If for some reason his hand slipped off, he had to go back and start over and touch the door knob just once.

Everything in his life now became these obsessive compulsive behaviors, so we have thought and emotion looking for safety through behaviors instead of thinking like it was before in the preparation. He says it was interesting because it shifted. In that first lifetime, it was about being prepared for disaster. I have to think ahead. I have to plan ahead. In this lifetime, it was everything right now safe because of this ritual — I wasn't thinking ahead.

Now he says that in that lifetime he pretty much drove himself and everybody else crazy. But it was a different kind of crazy. There was no recognition of insanity, it was a constant search of being safe, but it was always finding the little fix that was making it safe. He says that was an interesting lifetime because in his mind I didn't think of it as non-productive because every little thing that I figured out was a safety — a step forward in his mind because he got to feel safe with that one little thing.

I am very sure that you were creative (smile). *Oh my! He is showing rituals that are just so …!!*

He had a wife, he was male in this lifetime and she looked at it like it was her responsibility to make sure the nutty professor survived. And he set things up so that he could do his rituals and not lose his mind. So she supported him in that. He says in a way that was good because, otherwise, I would have been thrown in a "looney bin." I would have been in something like Bedlam. He says in a way it was bad because it supported my addiction. Jay says that it was really rough on her because she didn't know what ritual he was going to come up with for a new situation. She would watch for the signs and she got to the point where she could read him very, very, well.

Those are two key lifetimes that locked addiction in. There is a little bit more of the obsessive compulsive behaviors. He's laughing. I even had to die obsessive compulsive!

He is showing himself really, really ill. He is in bed and he had a ritual for making the bed, and one for how the blankets had to be folded over, and which pillows had to be in place. He says that while he is dying he is checking the rituals. The second he noticed all the rituals were in place and everything in the room is the way it is supposed to be with his wife beside the bed where she is supposed to be – death. It's safe now; I can go now.

The point I am making with these two lifetimes is addiction always goes to "I am not safe". **All addictions are based in "I am not safe."** He says that is really important for the healing of addictions. If we can find people's safety zone and help them into a safety zone in their own minds, there is no more addiction.

He is talking about first there was thought, now it is behavior and, of course, it's all tied in to emotions – the emotion of I am not safe. He says at that point we now push ourselves to where we can't find safety inside the mind even with the rituals, and that is where the outer stuff comes in.

Now we are going to go where he discovered a natural plant that took the edge off. And he says we are skipping a lot of lifetimes here – we are just going to the primary ones.

So he says, we are going to go to a lifetime where it's the equivalent of learning how to smoke pot. This was really more of a lifetime of hiding through plants. This has something to do with Hawaii a long, long time ago. He says do the equivalent of the native boy's mentality where if you do it, everything will be fine; if not, no need to worry, you will do it tomorrow. If it is not in place, no problem. He says he lived in a culture where they did not know it, but they were affected by the plants they were eating. There was something in the diet that was a relaxer and it became an almost sacred plant. They didn't know why it became a sacred plant. They thought it was a healing plant to not make you crazy.

He is showing it as being handed down through the generations. It was never thought of like we think of marijuana; it was thought of like this is a sacred plant that connects you (not to safety although that is the feeling) with the "All of Life" (the oneness of all). It makes you more of who you are. And it was in the diet; it wasn't smoked or anything, it was just part of the diet. And he is also showing some of the American native stuff where they had it. They didn't smoke it but they would drink or eat it. In that lifetime, children were introduced to it at a very young age – like putting it into a baby's formula because it was believed that it helped the individual stabilize and become accustomed to the physical world.

Again, we are going to go into rituals. There was a belief that the soul came into the body not fitting the physical world and you would use these food, plants, etc. So he says in this lifetime, it was not one of the "Yo Dude!" lifetimes. People were productive; they weren't frantic. They understood that time is irrelevant. He says that they may have taken it a little too far. In that lifetime, once again, he is a male. He did a lot of male lifetimes. We usually choose one gender over another for most of our learning. It appears he mostly chose male.

He is laughing. Yeah, I did it the hard way. What can I say?

He says that in this lifetime he was a family man again. Think of it as living in a culture less stressed than the American way of living. If something doesn't happen today, we will do it tomorrow. It was a lot like that. It was not a bad culture, it was not a lazy culture, it was an "easy does it" culture - time for living. He says the problem with that was the idea for time for living well got tied into the vibrational frequency of the plants. And emotionally, mentally, it got tied in with the "I need the plants to live this life" because that was the culture.

He says that was a pretty nice life.

12:21. He says, look at the clock quick – a 6. 6 means one completed cycle, another one started. It's also about moving into spirit. Two 2s – 2 is all about relationships. He says 12 is a Master number reverse the mirror. We are going to present the mirror to ourselves. So 12:21 now each of those is a 3 which is of course the trinity. He says that when it is presented in 2 threes it's about relationships.

He says this is specifically relationships of opposites in the physical, in this case opposite life styles because he is showing when he was probably around 28 years old, their culture was very isolated. It was a large culture, but it was very remote. There is something about an outside culture coming in and the outside culture was rigid, and it was very push, do, be, and be present. Now you have the mirror coming in as what is your lifestyle compared to someone else's. They had no comparisons before that.

And it was a shock that ran through the entire culture. He literally shows it like the A bomb. They had no concept of that existing in life and it was just there. The rest of life was hiding the plants because if the new culture found out where the "I'm okay" vibration was coming from that was keeping them from entering into the new culture, they would have destroyed them. By that time, they had become completely dependent on that way of life because they really thought it was the right way (kind, loving).

He says now we have addictions on all levels. We have the addiction of thought with the emotions that started the whole thing that is tied in with all the levels. Then, we have the thought addiction - I have to do this all the time, I have to think. Then, we have the obsessive compulsive of thought, but it now comes into behavior. The fear is always there. The "I am- not- safe fear" is always present in all addictions, always the root cause.

Coming into the plant addiction, I now need something outside of myself to be safe. It is not the behaviors; it is taking the vibrational frequency of something else. So now we have brought it to almost full completion because there has been implanted a belief that in order to get rid of the really crappy feelings, I need to ingest something. He says now we are going to tie it into a habitual vibrational frequency. We know it is missing, but we don't know what it is.

The vibrational frequency in the first life was I have to watch all the time so I will be safe. The second life was I have to do the rituals all the time to make sure everything is tightly controlled and specific, and I will be safe. The third life was that I have to ingest this plant, be part of a culture and I will be safe.

He says now we come into the lifetimes where we have all this embedded on all levels and we don't know what the hell we are doing. Now coming into this time period, because he has done this in other cycles, you are very well aware of the fact that it is considered an unstable frequency – we are in transition. What we call "good" is coming up big time; what we call "bad" is coming up big time. Everything is at risk because it is the transition.

*So he says, look at kids like me. We come into this lifetime where societal beliefs are in flux. The old stuff isn't right, the new stuff isn't right, and the old and new stuff are still battling with each other. **So I come into this lifetime, I have two purposes. One is to overcome; the other is to teach if I don't overcome**. He says that we are going to boil it down to that simple – of course, there are a lot of other purposes. He says now look at a kid like me. I am very empathic and I care very much, I want to do the right thing, I have no idea why I am afraid all the time. Now in this culture and time period, drugs are accepted by my peers. Drugs are the answer given to me and they are so easy to find - they are everywhere!*

Mom, I could have gotten them anywhere I went. I didn't need money.

There are barter systems and there are friends who will help you get high. Look at that lifetime when I lived where all were doing the plants. If a friend noticed that you were getting anxious or afraid, they would hand you a plant or hand you food with a plant in it or a drink, something, anything, because it was the right thing to do. He says that is what is happening in this culture.

Even though in this culture, the children know it is wrong because the adults say so, the children don't believe the adults. They flat out know the adults are wrong. He said this is one of the issues. The children come in knowing something is wrong and something has to fix it. The parents say that is not the right way to fix it but they don't give the way that works right away like the drugs do.

WHAT IS THE WAY THAT WOULD HAVE WORKED FOR YOU?

He is smiling and says there really wasn't one.

He says the right way is going to the basis of fear of non-survival, fear of death. I am not safe and he said that with everything that moved into place with this culture, we didn't have an instant fix. We have some of the fixes coming up that are a whole lot better than we used to have, a lot more understanding, but he says that is really the catch 22 here. The kids can find what they think is an instant fix in the drugs to the point where they don't care if it is going to hurt them later.

And they don't believe the adults. He says that part of the reason they don't believe them is that they are told that sex isn't good either. They are so wrong. He says look at all the pleasures of life the adults tell us is wrong and they can't give us a good reason; they can't give us a reason we can hang onto and know right now right here.

So he says that what is happening to addictions, more and more the understanding is coming in but there is going to be a recurring cycle of individuals who got caught in the addictions coming into the time periods where they are more understood.

And he says for him, this is a part of a formula. He was coming in this lifetime to hopefully overcome it. Quite frankly, he says, "I knew coming in there was a pretty good chance I wouldn't overcome it." So what he was doing was a stepping stone process, hoping to overcome addiction; if not, working with you to help others understand addiction. (Our plan). Now if you look at his peers, the message was "I died." He saying "Yo, dude, you moron. I died. Hello, wake up! This is a wake-up call."

WHEN YOU COME IN NEXT LIFETIME, WILL I BE WITH YOU THAT LIFETIME?

He just winked — you guys haven't decided yet. He says, at least part of it. It's very possible because you guys have been doing this work together for a very long time. He says that he is going to choose a female form next lifetime.

WHEN YOU DECIDE TO HAVE ANOTHER HUMAN EXPERIENCE, HOW WILL YOU DEAL WITH YOUR ADDICTIONS?

He is going to come back during a time when the methods that we use are more based in the energy of love, and in using that energy of love, it will be separated out into different methods where you use color, sound, and movements of the physical body where things are released or drawn in basically balanced that way. And doing that with the work he is doing now, it is expected that he will make a major break in that addiction cycle.

HOW WILL YOU KNOW WHOM TO CHOOSE TO SHARE THAT LIFETIME?

We are going to go into that whole reincarnation thing. He says, Yeah, I am going to make the pre-incarnation agreement like we always do, but the bottom line is that once you get there, you have free will. So there is a risk factor. He says the risk is much less that lifetime than this one because of the direction we are moving in our understanding in the physical right now.

However, he also says that coming into that lifetime, yes, he is going to carry this forward with him, there will be a little better understanding with himself of that feeling of not being safe, but once again, we are going to do the blue print, that is the outline. I am going to make the plan: this will be my mom, this will be my dad, my cousins, this is who I am going to meet and marry and all that stuff, but once you step into the body, free will asserts. He says it is always a risk.

Now the good news. He says we have to remember that even though he is talking about these physical lifetimes we work on this between lives as well. He says what is happening now no matter how many souls (hundreds of thousands) who were going through this cycle are now working the equivalent as frantically on the other side to create – think of it like an energy bridge – you are talking about the cellular memory, the DNA, all this good stuff, he says think of DNA at thought level, emotion, behavior spirit, all of it. It's all DNA. When you are on the other side, what you are doing is creating a bridge where you have access to activate the antidote.

THE ANTIDOTE BEING YOUR TIE TO YOUR HIGHER POWER?

That is the ultimate antidote, yes. Now when we go into the physical, we are going to look at the sub-antidotes. That would be activating a spark within self that says I want to go to this teacher. We use to think of them as coincidences. It is walking by a café that is advertising a two-hour coffee seminar type of thing that evening. And just for the heck of it, you decide to go. He says that is what helps you turn around. He says that it is all about finding the people who will help you find yourself and find God.

CAN YOU SHARE ANOTHER LIFETIME WITH US?

Sure. Looking to a lifetime where I was an adrenaline "junkie," an adventure "junkie." You name it and I did it. In that lifetime, I became addicted to the endorphin rush, and I had to have more and more, just like any addict. I started out doing little things like tempting the neighbor's dog to bite me. You would equate it with bungee jumping nowadays. It kept escalating.

I didn't like my life. It was boring and stressful and horrible. I hated it so I looked for an escape. The easier escape was escaping death. My addiction to life-threatening circumstances became my ability to feel life. That is a very, very slippery slope. It actually became tangled up within me that that kind of high is what it takes to feel alive. My real life became unreal. It all revolved around creating the next surge of adrenaline.

Now looking at it in this lifetime, I became addicted to those feelings. Drugs become the easiest way to create feelings artificially. Drugs are the easiest way to escape from the reality we don't want or don't like or are afraid of because it all boils down to the fear of being where, who, and what we are.

In this lifetime, (this addictive personality was started many lifetimes ago and has been going on many lifetimes) that need to step out of the human existence was part of the addiction. It had already been established. I knew beforehand that I probably would not be strong enough to beat the addiction in this lifetime so you and I set it up so where the win would be that I do beat the addictions or the win would be that I do not beat the addictions, I leave early and you and I spread the word to help others come out of it. Also with that comes a weakness.

He is smiling.

Looking at human life takes a great deal of courage. Even those we think of as being unaware who go to work, eat, sleep, play a little, and repeat that, have the courage to accept what is in that moment and handle it. All glory to them. But what happens when you start this kind of cycle, this kind of behavior (not the kind of behavior here but of the energetic system) is like the greyhound that is conditioned to chase the rabbit it will never get. That entire program is set up within the system. Just the opposite of the individual we think of as they aren't aware, they are just working, having a little fun, having a beer and going to sleep. We think of them as not being aware, but they are more aware than the ones who try to escape reality...more aware, more *courageous of where they are, more able to do what is right in front of them. They are not running away. So in this case they are actually doing the greater work than the one who runs away. We don't usually think of it that way.*

*Once again, looking at it as an entire energetic system, we say that this physical body is just a physical form. But it is **not** just a physical form. It is simply a condensation of all that we are into a human form so that we can experience all that we are, including addictive behaviors. So past lives can affect and create addiction in a trillion different ways. It can be a lifetime where there was so much fear that we brought it into our being with so much intensity that we are addicted to fear, and that addiction to it creates further addictions.*

It is so complex that it is not possible to put it into human volumes, but it is possible to put the basic understanding in it. And that is where we are going with it because that is where we will find the healing - that is where we will turn it around.

CAN YOU SHARE A HAPPY LIFETIME WITH US?

He says, let's look at a fun one. He is kind of rolling his eyes because he is going back to a lifetime when he was a female. He says he experimented with being a female.

In that lifetime, he had yellow blond hair in ringlets and he is in a very fancy dress, and whatever family he belonged to had everything they needed. We were not fabulously wealthy, but we had plenty and knew that we would always have plenty.

That is one of the major things that is missing in addictions (there is absolutely no concept of having plenty and always will have plenty – it is always dangerous in addiction).

In that lifetime, he was the adored little girl. He was in a family of Mom, Dad and three brothers. He was the last one to come along and she was the apple of everyone's eyes, as she was the only girl. It was very balanced, everyone did what they had to do and you weren't allowed to be a brat.

Jay is laughing and says I got away with it a little bit but he did that in this lifetime too.

So in that lifetime, she grew up on a great big, rambling farm somewhere over in France in a brick house, and brick walls located on sprawling rolling hills. Basically, she grew up in a paradise where she had her ponies, horses, dogs, cats, kittens, birds and all kinds of things. She had good friends she met at Sunday gatherings – it was a very simple life because the rules were very clear. You do unto to others as you would have them do unto you. You have and do your responsibilities to the best of your ability and you laugh and you love. Those were the main rules. It was very simple. So even though they had very nice things, there wasn't any ego about it. It wasn't showing off for the neighbors, it was appreciating what the creator provided; it was enjoying beauty. There was a great deal of appreciation of beauty.

In that lifetime, I had many teachers. Of course, I had my parents who were good people. My father was a little strict, but that was okay, it was in keeping. And I also had the teachings of my brothers because my brothers looked out for me. They were fiercely protective of me and I had to help them understand that I needed to learn on my own, but it was fun because they watched not out of fear but out of love, out of joy. They thought it was a blast.

They were quite a bit older than I was and thought it was a blast to play with this little doll. So I grew up with love and never a thought of fear. If fear reared its head, everyone was immediately brought back to the fact that there is a source. We didn't understand how it worked or why it worked, but they had absolute belief that it worked and so it did. No addiction that lifetime.

Jay laughed and said that you could say I was addicted to feeling good and having fun.

WAS THERE ADDICTION IN THE LIFETIME BEFORE THAT?

He represents it like a game of checkers. In this case, there were the times he would come in and addiction would be created, some would be lessened, like take two steps forward, one step back. Then, he might have a couple of lifetimes where it was pretty much downhill. Then, it gets to a certain point where you know you have to live a lifetime with less stress to assist yourself in being able to create a sense of safety while in the physical body. It's not a way we choose very often because we look at it as wasting time. We are in the human body and we want to work on this and correct that, etc. But in this case, creating that sense of safety and knowing while in the physical body was absolutely essential.

What was the addiction that became so strong that you easily carried it from one lifetime to another?

He is going to say six lifetimes, actually more like a dozen lifetimes ago, but if you wanted to find the absolute "hammer down" point where it was Ohhh, CRAP! It was about six lifetimes ago. In fact, you can say it became a major problem a lot of lifetimes ago.

And what created it, besides fear?

It's a continuation of learned behaviors seeking to feel better because of judgments saying, I don't feel good now. I judge things as right or wrong, and they are what I want or what I don't want. This is a KEY POINT in addiction. We judge something as what we want or don't want, which is what we call good or bad, and we can become addicted to judging things to the point of where unless it is absolutely perfect and making us feel marvelous, it's bad. No gray area. It's either what I want and I am happy and, of course, what I want is based on a preconceived notion of what I think will make me happy or it's not what I want and, therefore, it is bad, bad, bad and must be escaped from.

Say, for example, you come into a normal lifetime, it's a work-a-day world, like the guy we talked about earlier where we thought of him as unaware, but who is actually more aware than the one who tries to escape. He does his duty as presented to him, does the best he can, sleeps, eats, drinks, works and that's it - his whole lifetime.

So coming into a lifetime like that if you are in the cycle of chasing what you think will make you happy, judging everything as good or bad and, of course, that judging is based on will that make me feel happy or does it not make me feel happy. If you come into a lifetime like that, and you are predisposed to that, you are going to take a negative outlook on everything in your life. If someone gives you a flower and says "I love you," you might be so steeped in the negativity of the fact that you are doing the dishes that you don't even notice the beauty of the flower and the saying I love you.

SO IN THIS LIFETIME WHERE YOU KNEW YOU WERE IN TROUBLE, WAS THERE ANYTHING OUT OF THE ORDINARY? WAS THERE WAR? AN ACCIDENT WHERE YOU WERE SICK AND NEEDED SOMETHING TO EASE THE PAIN OR WAS IT FEELINGS?

*All. But the feelings are the foundation of everything you just said. But all of these experiences have been his. There was World War I where he was injured, and he keeps showing morphine, one of those that make you crazy. It kills the pain, but you go nuts. And it has been things like physical problems, deformities, injuries, illnesses – all of these. He says now look at it from the other side because all of these I was experiencing were circumstances I drew to myself through the negativity of my addiction. It is a vicious cycle. It's my own creation. He is firm on this. **He says addiction is created by self and no one else** and once people come to that understanding, then they can come to the understanding that they have absolute power to turn that around.*

We talked about once we get addicted, the physical body needs this, and needs that, which puts us into a position of helplessness. We have to understand that it is NOT helplessness. WE have absolute control over the physical body; we just have to find the way to do it.

JAY, DID YOU LIVE LIFETIMES IN WAR?

Yes. There were hundreds of lifetimes dealing with addiction. He picked out the four that would be the clearest examples and different stages. He says, imagine this level of addiction (I am talking about the lifetime where I am locked into survival) happens ten times. Then next lifetime, it happens 3 or 30 times. We are talking about one lifetime compared to thousands and that strain goes through. You will be in a lifetime where you make some headway against it, then, you will be in one where you don't.

Like this lifetime for him, he made major headway against it. It may not look like it, but he did. You already know that. The wars that you are talking about, he says, some of those were things like that culture with the plants — they were very laid back and loving — and the new culture came in. That was war over about 200 years and he was in two different bodies that lifetime of war. At first it wasn't an overt war, it was just that censorship. The new culture comes in and says there is something wrong with you and we are going to show you a better way. You are like children who need to be taught.

Jay says that is as bad as warfare. It's just not as obvious.

But he has lived different lifetimes where you can call it war. Look at it like American Indians. They didn't call it war, but they fought against different tribes all the time. They were constantly attacking each other. He says, I've had a lot of lifetimes where it wasn't declared war, but it was constant war. And it was okay because it was honorable. He says he was in World War I, by the way.

I WAS TOLD ONCE THAT YOU HAD BEEN IN VIETNAM. WERE YOU IN THE VIETNAM WAR?

No, but his energy is tied very close to it, though. You know that the Vietnam veterans are all going through issues we haven't seen in the other wars. It ties in directly with chemical addictions. Vietnam was the first time we did major biochemical warfare, at least in this cycle of the earth. Look at the addictions that he was talking about — mental, emotional, and behavioral — all this good stuff.

He says, my vibrational frequency is very similar to the Vietnam Vet. In that sense, he was one of them. You would find the energies merging together like this. I wasn't in it physically. So he has the vibrational frequencies that match because of the bio-chemical warfare. He was also doing a lot of work on it from the other side because he knew what was going to happen with the chemicals being released that would have an effect with the ones who already have the vibrational frequency of the chemicals.

This is going so many levels.

The way he is showing it is the whole tapestry that says this is what we are doing on the earth plane now, this is how it ties into the past, and this is how it is going to help us destroy or create the world. The Vietnam War was one of the key points because of what we were doing.

He says, it started a long time ago; we just didn't know about it. He says this is the first time it was open in 80% of the war. He says, we are now still feeling the vibrational frequencies of that, and that is one of the things they are really trying to reverse. Post-Traumatic Stress Syndrome is partly from the emotional impact of where they were, and part of it is the vibrational frequencies of the chemicals.

He says, think of sound. The sound of battle, then silence, means someone is creeping up on you. All sounds become threatening and, once again, remember at the seat of addiction is fear.

Let's look again at energy, knowing that everything is energy - our thoughts, words and actions. Once we create via any of those three things, that creation, that energy, remains even if to a lesser degree or until it is replaced with a higher frequency.

THANK YOU. LOVE YOU.

Love you, too.

Where there is love, there is healing.

CHAPTER 5

WHERE DOES ADDICTION LIVE?

We all have addictions whether they are the more accepted; addiction to sugar or coffee or the harsher ones of drugs and alcohol or others. In order to live WITHOUT ADDICTION NOW we first need to look at and understand where addiction lives and thrives – in what part of us.

I remember Jay saying many times that our society is outward focused and we are consistently measuring ourselves and others by what they *do* which is a form of living outside ourselves. So if I speak about living inward, what does that mean?

What I am talking about is getting in touch with your "inner knowings" that exist in each one of us and is a part of our soul that knows how to live to the highest in all ways.

"Living inward" doesn't mean that you withdraw from society or you become reclusive or exclusive; it means that you take what you know that serves society well, and extend that into living fully and completely, participating 100% in our outward focused society, and make that work for you. In other words, living inward simply means coming from the inside to the outside of self and sharing that way of living with yourself and others. It is a loving, healthy way to live in balance.

However, there are some things that can block you from doing this. And one of them is one of the greatest deterrents to success for anyone addicted (or not) and is the "monkey chatter" that we all have. 90% of our population has an addiction to that part of the mind where "monkey chatter" exists – that self-talk that is in contrast to peace, calm, and positive thoughts.

Jay says that this was so difficult for him because the chatter within his mind seemed to never stop and "monkey chatter" is *always* negative. It tells you all the things that you are doing or have done are wrong, wrong, wrong – that you should have, shouldn't have, should do, shouldn't do, etc. And it seems to never shut up. And it won't until you learn how the higher and lower minds work so that you can "quiet" your mind and stop the "monkey chatter" and become closer to living without addiction.

JAY, CAN YOU HELP EXPLAIN THIS?

Let's talk about quieting the mind . . . so many people have become completely confused on what that means. They believe that the mind is the self - that the mind is divine mind rather than individual mind. They get confused on what is logic and what is the higher intelligence. They don't understand that logic is a function of the physical form and a function of the formulas that is created to exist in the physical plane with the rules that we have here.

Logic is simply a tool that we use by (we are going to use the phrase the lower mind) simply to compare it to high intelligence - so basically what we are doing is saying the formulaic mind of the physical world we are going to call the lower mind. The high intelligence cosmic wisdom we will call divine mind or higher mind. It is not that one is better than the other, it is that they are supposed to be serving different functions.

But what has happened is that the lower mind has been perceived as the God, the wisdom here in the physical. The lower mind is the false God.

I AM CALLING THE LOWER MIND THE "MONKEY CHATTER," IS THAT RIGHT?

Yeah, that is what we are talking about because most people's lower minds have been taken over by the "monkey chatter." It's all negative. And they haven't come to understand that that has to be completely released.

Right now what they are doing as a fix is gaining what they think of as control over the lower mind by doing things as logical formulas. They will work crossword puzzles, they will organize a closet, they will read a book or they will watch television. They think it is quieting the "monkey chatter" when really what it is doing is giving the mind something else to do. That's all. The mind is still in control — it still gets to do what it wants to do so that many of the people are being fooled thinking quieting the mind means giving it something logical to do because it is soothing to look at cross word puzzles and say, "Oh goody. I have it done; I have a sense of accomplishment; I am intelligent, and everything fits in the right place and the lower mind is happy."

People think that the lower mind is quiet and they don't even have a concept of accessing the higher mind or the peace and quiet within self. So a lot of people don't understand the difference or do not understand what it means when you say "quiet the monkey chatter." They think you are saying finding some kind of peace and accomplishment through using that same mind for solving different problems set up specifically so that the mind has something to do.

SO TO QUIET THE MIND AND THE MONKEY CHATTER, IT IS REALLY THROUGH MEDITATION?

It is. And another issue that you have noticed over and over again is that so many are under the control of the "monkey chatter" that they can't seem to find a way to escape it. It's like a blind man in a room without any doors or windows. He can feel the walls all he wants, but he is going to stay in that room. He is trying to use the same lower mind to get out of the "monkey chatter" and you can't do that. Again, that is why they go into crossword puzzles, watching TV, reading a book, whatever it is. They don't realize that all they are doing is giving the lower mind something else to do to make them feel better.

That is why there are steps required to clear that "monkey chatter" and, of course, that is why the steps are going to be different for each individual. Each individual is in a different position.

Meditation where you sit quietly, close your eyes and clear your mind of any thoughts, allowing you to find the truth of your reality is the highest form that we have found in the physical plane to this point as meditation is understood now. And many people do have to take the stepping stones and some of that is a simple sit-down and admit to their self that their lower mind runs the show and is tricking them. Many people will not admit that.

They like to think that watching television and reading a book or working a crossword puzzle is them taking control of their mind. It isn't.

So, in this case, like with addictions, admission is the first step – admission and recognition or recognition followed by admission. And that, of course, is hinged on them understanding the difference.

So many people have not felt what you termed the peace and the calm. They have a vague theoretical knowledge of it at best, but it has no reality for them. 90% of the population is in addiction of the mind now and is one of the reasons that upheaval is so great.

One of the first things that can be done is to sit down and explain the differences between the lower mind and the higher mind, and that would have to be explaining what lower mind is and what higher mind is and what it does and doesn't do for each.

WHAT IS A SIMPLER WAY TO EXPLAIN THE DIFFERENCE BETWEEN THE LOWER AND HIGHER MIND?

Okay. Let's look at the purposes between the two. The lower mind is really not the lower mind at all. It is an aspect of intelligence that is created to be able to associate and create formulas for easier living while in the physical body. It is just an aspect of creation, mind and intelligence - whatever you want to call it. Its sole purpose is to function under the guidance and command of the higher mind or divine intelligence and to be used as a tool to be recognizing and associating.

For example, the mind should be the one that says "Oh, the last time I touched my finger to the fire it hurt. I won't do that again." And that should be the extent of its power. It is basically a survivor tool that has been given the power and authority to be in command of the entire life.

Higher mind or divine mind is that aspect of oneness that is the creative intelligence that exists in every single thing created and uncreated. It is the "all-ness," the knowing — think of it as the complete synchronicity of life with its self. That is what it is supposed to be - in command, running the show with the lower mind.

So once people understand that, they can look at the lower mind and say, "All right, but I have it under control because I can do crossword puzzles, I can feel better about this"…that and the other thing. But they will come to understand the lower mind has no connection with the rest of the world. It is extremely isolated. Lower mind is all about survival. It is also all about separation.

AND THAT IS WHERE THE ADDICTS GET CAUGHT, ISN'T IT?

Yes. And as you have pointed out many times, there are so many kinds of addicts. Right now our greatest addiction problem is the mind — the lower mind. And that greatest addiction is a key element in what you were talking about earlier in hiding in alcohol, drugs and excessive behaviors of any kind, and excessive thoughts of any kind. It all ties in with the lower mind. It is all about separatism. Of course, that is the fear you are talking about.

If we are separate, we have everything to fear. If we are in higher mind or divine mind, we have nothing to fear. We are one with everything. Everyone is our brother, sister and loved one, including storms that comes up on the horizon.

So once people understand that there are two different aspects of creation with two very different intended purposes, they see what has happened is that the lower mind has fooled them into thinking they have control. If they had control, they would be able to feel peace and calm at any given moment. That is the key element. If they can't feel peace and calm at any moment, they are not in control of the lower mind. They must understand the difference between peace and calm and just feeling a sense of satisfaction or accomplishment. There is a huge difference.

MOST OF THE TIME, I AM LIVING IN PEACE AND CALM AND DO NOT WORRY ABOUT MUCH ANYMORE, AND IN ESSENCE HAVE BECOME THE OBSERVER OF LIFE. HOW DID I ARRIVE AT THAT WITH THE LOWER MIND?

You have used a couple of different methods over and over again. First of all, you used grief. You used the process of sorting out your experiences to look for a sense of what is beyond the actual experiences. The lower mind looks only at the experience. Because you have a faith in something greater than this individualized aspect of creation that we call ourselves, you looked beyond what is there right in front of your eyes, your nose and your toes, as they say. And because of that, you expanded your faith – expansion in the sense of expanding peace, calm, wisdom, all that good stuff. That is one of the major tools you used.

And the second you used is the chakra work you do with clearing out the energy pockets. As you know, clearing out the energy pockets is clearing out body, mind and emotions, which is, of course, soul because soul is everything. [Refer to Joan's three previous books regarding the seven major chakras.]

The third that you used is meditation. So you used a three-fold plan and worked diligently at it to recognize the difference between the lower mind and the higher mind or the physical mind and the divine mind. That is one of the key elements that you did, saying that you watch life and have become the observer because you recognized there is a difference which is a key element.

PEOPLE TALK ABOUT THE BODY, MIND AND SPIRIT AND YOU TALKED ABOUT THE HIGHER MIND WHICH SOUNDED AS IF IT IS SPIRIT. SO WHAT IS THE DIFFERENCE BETWEEN THE HIGHER MIND AND THE SPIRIT?

There isn't any, really, although people are labeling them differently. Higher mind is the aspect that we would think of as divine intelligence of the soul or spirit. That's all. It's all the same thing. It is creative power; it is God; it is divine mind, divine intelligence; universal wisdom - whatever you want to call it. However, it is being labeled and defined differently by some people. If you are talking about Spirit with a capital S as within the spirit that is all aligned, divine mind is an aspect of that.

BESIDES WHAT I HAVE DONE, WHAT ARE THE OTHER STEPS TO BRING THE LOWER MIND TO THE CONNECTION OF SOURCE?

First and foremost, the individual needs to be at a point where they are willing to admit they do not have command over their life. It is not just command over the lower mind. If you don't have command over the "monkey chatter," and you can't shut it off, then you have NO command over your life anywhere. You know how in many recovery programs you are told to surrender, that you have no control, just give it up, and just let it go. Well, it's the same thing with individuals in any walk of life, including those that are addicted to the "monkey chatter" or the drama or the emotions or any of those obsessives. They have to reach that point where they are willing to give up the idea, the illusion that they are in control of their lives and until that happens they don't move forward.

Of course, they can work on getting there, absolutely. For example, you did that. It took you many steps to come to the realization of the objective observer because you were willing to do that.

Bottom line: anyone who is in any kind of addiction, the most important thing for them is to question their own faith because those who are in the addiction of "monkey chatter" (lower mind) have faith only in the physical, only in the separatism. They don't have any real faith to hang onto. When you are controlled by the "monkey chatter" it is all isolation and separatism.

We would recommend that they start exploring what they DO believe in instead of touting what they don't believe in. Exploring who they really are, and where their power comes from. See that is the key issue. They need to understand where their power really comes from.

WE KNOW THAT YOU (JAY) ARE PLANNING TO REINCARNATE AGAIN, SO WHAT HAVE YOU BEEN WORKING ON SO WHEN YOU COME IN YOU WILL LOOK AT LIFE DIFFERENTLY? WHAT ARE YOU DOING ON THE OTHER SIDE?

First and foremost, I am, I guess you would call it, taking a course in the Absolute, in the love that maintains and holds complete under all circumstances no matter what is going on. You might think of it as what we think of as the difference of the father energy and the mother energy. I discovered after getting here that I didn't have any kind of a concept of that Absolute love that just simply holds in place with no judgment. There isn't even a concept of judgment here. And I realized that my entire energy needs to be infused with that as much as possible before I incarnate again. So I am taking courses in not intellectually understanding but incorporating and accepting those kinds of energies – the Oneness.

I am also looking at the thought patterns that are prevalent on the earth plane right now. There are so many of them, but you can boil it down to five or six that are dominating everything that is going on. I am working with the higher teachers to understand these thought patterns, to take them back to their root cause in order to assist in healing that energy. And at the same time, to be able to heal in the physical form when I take that physical form.

What are those thought patterns?

First and foremost, what you have brought up many times is the thought pattern that no one loves me, no one understands me. It is a separation. That is what the separation is and the isolation boils down to — no one loves me, no one understands me, no one is going to help me. That is the original mistake, forgetting who we are. So everything boils down to we forgot who we are, and then we compounded the injury by rejecting who we are when it was represented to us. We didn't believe it.

Another thought form is that we are only here for a short time. We must get everything we can and we must do everything we can because we are only here once; we only have one shot. This has proven to be extremely harmful to all life forms here on the earth plane.

Another basic belief is that we have to find our happiness through someone else or something else. It points back to what you were saying about an outwardly focused world. Most of us are taught from the time that we are born that approval by society and having this, that, and the other thing in our lives are the only real measures of whether or not we are good people. And every culture does this to one degree or another. Of course, you can see it very clearly in western cultures.

Another underlying thought is the fear of love. The fear of love exists because there is a certainty deep inside that it will be taken away. This relates directly back to we knew who we were, we knew the oneness, we WERE love and we lost it.

So these are some of the most destructive and the most dominant or pre-eminent thought forms on the earth plane right now. And if you trace them back you see that they all go back to the feeling abandoned and lost. We are covering a deep pain, a still open wound.

I AM SO HAPPY AND EXCITED FOR YOU, JAY, AND WHAT YOU ARE LEARNING.

He is representing it as absolutely fascinating. And he is so hopeful – he is so gung ho. He is saying, we can do this; I know we can do this.

If it is okay, he wants to talk about the thought forms that are being projected to the earth plane right now that are also being projected from individuals in the human form that are the opposite of the destructive thoughts. He wants to give you some good news!

He is looking at the earth plane – he is showing pockets of energy all through the earth plane. It is like lights coming on, and I can also see little lights coming on in individuals. He says that there has been a planting – it is kind of like planting people inside a corporation to change it from the inside, and it is individuals who have reached a point where they are ready to open to the truth that was lost in the first place – that there is more, that we are all connected, and they are on every level of being open to that truth whether it is just a kind of poking your toe in the water and saying, "Oh wow! That feels kind of good." or whether it is diving in head first. They are all over the planet.

The KEY to this is each one is at the space of opening up to being an active participant in love and in Oneness, and faith and hope. They are all over the place, and the thought form that is dominant on that side of the scale is I AM one. I AM loved. I AM all, which boils down to I AM. It is individuals in the physical form, and it is also individuals from all the known universe and unknown universe who are beaming it in with careful doses (you don't want to explode the place).

But beaming in careful doses is what Jay is showing as an energy coming in from the time we were created and is the actual pure memory of being in the God energy or being the God energy. He says THAT is what is waking up our planet earth now.

WOW! WHAT ARE SOME WAYS TO FORGIVE OURSELVES AND HEAL?

Loving and forgiving ourselves becomes so hard because that is where we never get to the point where we believe that we have no control over our lives. We always have the thought that I could have done better, I should have done better, I would have done better, blah, blah, blah. All of that is based in the thought I had control.

WE THINK THAT BECAUSE WE TELL EVERYBODY THAT WE CREATE WHAT WE HAVE.

Exactly, and there is insufficient understanding of the power of that creation and how it works through the body, mind, emotion. So one of the key elements people would look for is how do they as individualized aspects of the "One" process through the mechanism we have set up (an incredibly intricate mechanism) of what we call emotions, thoughts, body, all of that stuff. What are the filters in there and how does it process? People need to find out how they work — what makes them tick. Most people are afraid to do that.

WELL, ARE THERE CERTAIN STEPS? WHAT HAS WORKED FOR YOU JAY?

He is laughing. He said not much worked.

He is saying the influence of one that came from a higher vibration. He is showing a lifetime where he is on a desperate search to try to find a way out of some trouble he had gotten himself into through his addictive thoughts and behaviors. And in that lifetime, he would have called it a pure stroke of luck that he literally stumbled into and fell into a guy that was a higher teacher. He was a very humble individual, but his vibrational frequencies were so high that just being around him helped Jay pick himself up. And he says that if people are willing to start a path of finding their own meaning in life that can happen to anyone. The problem is because people are so mind-controlled they accept false teachers and they can't tell the difference.

He says in that lifetime the key for him was that he got so desperate that he would look anywhere for help in places that he hadn't already — he had already looked into addictions, all the people who believed in addictions, who shared them with him and all that good stuff and he just kept going down the toilet. And finally, he decided to look in a different direction because there was no more to explore on the dark side. He says that is the good news about hitting rock bottom; the bad news is you hit rock bottom and you can hurt a lot of people on the way.

And he says it is KEY now that some people who are stuck in addiction will not allow themselves to get to rock bottom. They will look at it and say, you know what? I just can't stand me anymore; I need to find a different me. And that is what you were talking about when you said you were becoming the objective observer. It is the same thing. You begin to wonder — who is that with the "monkey chatter" — where is that coming from? As you said, we can go into past lives, we can go into current life regression and see who it is that taught us the "monkey chatter."

And in that sense, we can go into forgiveness and all of this good stuff. But the bottom line is we must see where we bring it in and allow it to continue to control. Everyone is in control of whether or not the mind continues to control. You just don't know it.

SO IN FORGIVING YOU REALLY HAVE TO LOOK AT WHAT NEEDS FORGIVENESS, WHAT YOU HAVE DONE THAT YOU HAVE NOT LIKED AND ADDRESS THOSE ISSUES BY SURROUNDING IT WITH LOVE AND SENDING IT INTO THE UNIVERSE?

Yeah, show compassion for yourself. It's like facing demons. You know, little kids see the boogey man in the closet and the child goes up and faces it and sees it is just a shadow of a coat sleeve and the boogey man disappears. Those in addiction are hiding from their own boogey man — those things about themselves they don't like. So when you face it, it disappears if you let it.

Of course, then we get into the subject of guilt. Remember talking about the dominant thought patterns — guilt is one of them. Guilt has been used to manipulate for so many eons, it is now built into the thought system here on the earth plane. When we come to recognize a mistake that we made that we think of as a mistake, guilt usually takes over and does not allow for forgiveness.

So basically what is happening is a dominant thought form is coming in to keep that feeling of having done wrong in place to maintain the status quo – to maintain that feeling of separation. If you did something wrong, you are separated and not one of the whole; you are judged and condemned. And your own mind is the one judging and condemning you because your own mind is a part of that guilt platform. That is why it is so important for people to just give up on the idea of being in control. That way they can find a way to be in command.

When they talk about "give up," they are talking about giving up the old way of life, the "monkey chatter" which is the lower mind in control, giving up thinking you are in control when you are not – just giving up the old way.

IT IS SO MUCH EASIER WHEN YOU GIVE UP AND JUST LET BE, ISN'T IT?

Then you understand the balance of being able to do whatever you need to do of stepping up to the plate, clearing out whatever crap you need to but you do it with a sense of peace instead of a sense of desperation.

IT'S IMPORTANT TO BE WITH PEOPLE OF LIKE MIND, TOO. ISN'T IT?

Support groups are one way of being with people of like mind. It is absolutely essential that those people of like mind be on a positive level - not I give up, there is nothing I can do, oh woe is me. Rather the thinking of I give up the old way and by golly, I am going to grab the new way by the horns and ride the bull. That is why a lot of the recovery programs have trouble with re-occurring addictions.

Jay just said most of our recovery programs on our planet right now are based on the guilt platform. You recognize that you did wrong and you try to atone for it. That is not forgiveness. That is saying I did wrong now I have to do something to make up for it. And, he says, most of the recovery programs at the time they were started that is where their thought forms were and that was the best way to do it at that time, but we needed to come out of that at least 50 to 100 years ago and we didn't. Well, some of them are trying.

He is showing Hi, I am so and so, I am an alcoholic, I am a drug addict, whatever it is. He says, acknowledging and admitting is one of the first steps, but you can't stay at the first step and take the 20th. There has to come a time when you let that go. I AM is the most powerful, creative statement we make. Every time we say I AM an addict we are reinforcing that belief within our system. So that needs to be a fairly short time period when they are saying that.

If we could actually reach the point of forgiveness, then that wouldn't even be a true sense anymore except as a part of a learning experience we went through.

He says that it is interesting that in our cultures here on the earth plane, atonement has nothing to do with forgiveness because there is a belief that you can never do enough to earn it. And as long as it is felt that forgiveness has to be earned, it cannot be received. And people need to remember that when others say you have to forgive yourself, you cannot earn that forgiveness. You have to give it as a gift or you accept it as a gift.

You can forgive yourself; you don't need it from someone else, right?

Absolutely. In fact, you are the only one who can give it to yourself. If someone else does and you don't, it is not done. One of the biggest problems right now is that they don't understand what forgiveness is.

How do you define forgiveness?

Forgiveness is moving into an innocent perception. It is realizing that all mistakes made came out of its innocence in the sense that we did not know the harm we were causing. Even if we did it deliberately in a lifetime, we did not know what kind of harm we were causing because we felt we were isolated. Even the most heinous crime has a degree of innocence in it simply because it is created in the sense of separatism rather than in the sense of truth. We would think of it as a garbled way of looking at it but they say it is the truth.

Innocent perception is the knowing that everything that is done is based on a truth that is in place at that time. It is whatever that individual believed to be true, and in that sense, they are innocent. It may not be easy to see, but there it is. Look at yourself as an ax murderer in a lifetime and you were was pretty good at it.

If you looked at it now, you would go, "Oh my God!" You would be absolutely horrified. If you looked at the truth, you would feel nothing but compassion for that individual who was in so much pain and delusion that that was the only way he could find to express it. So if we look at our self in truth and compassion, we will just let it go.

Jay says that forgiving self is one of the biggest problems right now with that whole guilt thought form and, of course, the separation, and those that say I have sinned against God (we are taught that God exacts retribution).

Jay says there are no sins. There is what you might think of as mistakes, so get over it and don't do it again. That is how simple forgiveness should be – we recognize it, we don't like it, we forgive ourselves, we get over it and we just don't do it again.

SO UNDERSTANDING WHERE ADDICTION LIVES CAN HELP SIMPLIFY THINGS CAN'T IT?

Yes. Also, visualization is a great way to create illusion and when you create illusion, you can create your own reality. **If you visualize your addiction in the lower mind and see it moving up into the higher mind where addiction can't exist, you can clearly see your way out of addiction.** *Of course, there are things for you to do and states of being that help to move your addiction up into that higher mind.*

Remember, when you love yourself as part of the Oneness of All That Is, you give yourself permission to accept and honor all of the positive that is you without judgment of any thoughts or actions that you created in the past that were not to your highest good or the highest good of all. God does not judge but is only in appreciation for experiencing your choices and remains full of love for each one of us. And he wants you to know that in the whole of your being – in your soul.

REMEMBER: when you change your addiction from the lower mind to the higher mind you are actually changing from the conscious mind to the subconscious mind that gives the final approval or disapproval for your actions. The conscious mind can't see more than what it knows and is involved with logic and reasoning. The subconscious mind is where the emotions and stored memories (wisdom) lives so in order **to live without addiction, both your lower and higher mind must be in agreement or it will never happen**.

WHAT IS THE EASIEST WAY TO GET TO THE HIGHER DIMENSION?

The only way to get to the higher dimension is by increasing the love. That's it. If anyone wants a really, really simple formula, the only way or the smartest, easiest way is by activating more love in your life, more love in your being. That's the short cut.

I say it truly that when you go to the other side the only thing that you will really care about is how much love you felt and how much love you showed. It will be your only concern. All you have to do is remove the obstacles to your being loving– loving yourself and loving others. Remember, you can only love others to the degree that you love yourself.

THANK YOU. LOVE YOU.

Love you, too.

Where there is love, there is healing.

CHAPTER 6

COULD THIS BE ME?

We are all good people living the human experience, and because we all are human, we can complicate our lives through the emotion of fear and the freedom of choice or free will. Often, when we read about other people's addictions, we seem to think of those people as not like us and we can't fathom how they got to where they are.

By concentrating on Jay's addictions, it is easy to step away from appreciating how easy it is for any of us to get caught up in addiction. So let's explore two different scenarios of good, ordinary people who are trying their best to have success in their life. They might easily be us making poor choices in our living that create our own addiction(s) – all through free will.

Why is this beneficial to you? By reading their stories, we have the opportunity to see two entirely different people in different stages of their lives have similar experiences and feelings created by their addiction, caused by fear. We will *experience* how easy it is to begin a downward spiral when we look outside ourselves and our higher mind ways of living. And we can then see what Jay has to share with us about them.

These stories are not unique. Things like this happen all the time. It is only by being aware of what is happening around us and sending the love energy out to those that are caught in addiction that we can assist in overcoming addiction. When doing that, we are the *hope* to raise the earth's vibration that brings forth love, joy and peace in the world.

Does this sound simple? It is ... and it isn't.

SCENARIO 1

Let's pretend that we are a female 19 years of age who is attending college at the expense of her parents, who have saved for many years to put her through school, wanting her to have more in life than they had. Her family's economic situation could have afforded her a major scholarship, but at the end of her junior year in high school, she met someone who was in the "popular" group who became her boyfriend. This was a huge deal for her since she was shy and introverted.

In her senior year, her grades began to slip a little and she ended up with a much lower scholarship than they all had hoped for, which meant that she would be working part-time in the cafeteria serving food during mealtime as part of her scholarship agreement. She was angry at the college for at one point they had intimated that she might even be able to earn a full scholarship.

Heck! It wasn't her fault she was so busy in high school. Everyone kept stressing how important it was to have a social life outside of school for that helped round out your life, didn't it? And what was this deal in the kitchen? Serving food was not her idea of what college was meant to be about anyway. In addition to school work, it was a good time with lots of dates – that is what her friends kept telling her. Supposedly, the best time in her life is what her parents had told her.

Guys thought she was beautiful and told her so many times, making Saturday night fun at college a non-issue. And as her weekends began to fill up, they also began to consume much of her time and energy.

At the parties, she was lucky though because in spite of her not having extra money, all of her new friends were generous with her. The guys that were attracted to her had money enough to buy "party favors" for those party nights when all the "in crowd" swallowed pills, sipped a few drinks and ended up in bed for a little more fun.

At first, she had been hesitant to swallow anything she wasn't sure about, but what the heck? She and her old boyfriend in high school had smoked marijuana and that hadn't done that much. Made her sleepy is all. Besides, she was tired of being teased for being such a prude and wanted to fit in. And her beauty paid off for the guys always threw a few "crumbs" her way, a few leftovers from their own party favors. She loved the feeling she got with the drugs – she felt so sexy, powerful and free – just like her girlfriends. And if need be, in order to get the drugs, she had reached the point where she was willing to accommodate them sexually. This was nothing she thought she would ever do, but she liked being part of the group and had gotten to the point where she was becoming dependent on the drugs. It was already hard to get though the day without something.

Sure, she was aware that she needed to be careful not to get pregnant, but pills took care of that. And what was the big deal anyway? Everyone was doing it and her parents would never find out. So life went on but it was beginning to take a toll, especially after her first year at college. Things began to get more and more out of control. What was she to do?

It became harder and harder to concentrate and get all her work done on time especially since her scholarship work demanded her time at what now seemed to be awkward hours. She had already been called down to her school counselor to discuss her lack of progress in some of her classes. As much as she complained that the teachers expected too much from her, she only got a stern "buckle down now before it is too late" from her guidance counselor.

School break was coming and she would soon be headed home for Christmas holidays and, truly, she didn't want to disappoint her parents yet again. She loved them and knew that they had sacrificed for her. So she really concentrated for the next few days to do her best. But then, her new boyfriend from one of the top fraternities on campus called and said that he had a special holiday gift for her and asked if she could meet him that night? Without hesitating, she agreed for he was a "real catch," according to most of the females on campus.

She hopped into his waiting car and was surprised that he seemed angry. He said nothing and when she bent to kiss him, he just sat straight and firm in his seat and made no effort to meet her warm kiss. She sat back and said nothing. As he drove away, she asked him where they were going. He replied that they were going to meet some friends of his. She didn't ask anything more because it appeared that he might be high on something and she didn't want to aggravate him. She had learned that lesson the hard way earlier that month.

They arrived at a house off campus and she was relieved to see a few girl friends that she knew. They greeted her warmly and warned her that her boyfriend was out of sorts about the fact that she had slept with another of their friends to get drugs the other night. She would have to talk to him and explain that that had been the only way she could have gotten the drugs she needed and, at that point, she would have slept with King Kong if need be! He should understand for he had been the one to start her on cocaine.

She got a drink and a joint and headed his way where she saw him laughing, seeming much calmer. He grabbed her around the waist, stuffed a pill into her mouth and pulled her close to him covering her mouth with his and bit her lower lip hard until she swallowed the pill. She squealed and pushed him away. He laughed and took her hand and led her into one of the bedrooms. When he opened the door she was astonished to see several of his male friends in the room, though she was having trouble focusing on them for everything was becoming blurry. The last thing that she remembered was her boyfriend calling her terrible names and saying to his friends, "She is all yours. Have fun. Maybe this will teach her not to cheat on me."

When she woke many hours later, she was nude outside on the back lawn, bleeding between her legs. The more she became conscious, the more the pain travelled up her body, causing her to shiver. She couldn't understand what had happened and why she would be alone, naked in the backyard of a strange house. She got up on one elbow and called for help. No one answered.

She literally crawled on all fours to the back porch, opened the door and looked in. Bodies were sprawled all around the house with people passed out from booze, drugs or both. The pain is the only thing that kept her focused on getting her clothes and getting out of there. She finally found them and struggled to put them on. She knelt down beside one of the girls she knew and shook her awake and with whispers pleaded with her to drive her back to her dorm. After seeing her bruised and bleeding lips and cramped position, her girlfriend helped her to the car and announced that she was taking her to the emergency room at the local hospital, instead. She was too weak to argue.

At the hospital, the nurses took one look at her and warned her that there were others in front of her and they would get to her when they could. They asked her for her insurance card and were miffed that she didn't have that information with her. In fact, she had no idea where her purse was. Her girlfriend tried to reason with the nurses that it was very important that they admit her because she was bleeding profusely. Finally, one of them got up out of her seat and came forward. She led her into a curtained room and after a quick exam, called for a specialist. When the nurse returned, the girlfriend had left.

She used to be able to look into the mirror and see a sweet-looking, attractive enough girl with light brown mid-length hair and hazel eyes — never seeing the real beauty that others saw in her. Now as she peeked into the reflective glass, she couldn't believe what was looking back at her! Not even who, but what! She began to cry. How was this possible?

She was just an ordinary girl with high hopes of success in this world by following a path that many accomplished by attending college, getting good grades and creating options for a favorable future. All she had wanted was to be accepted by her peers and to be able to fit in.

Yet, here she was at the end of a long journey that had spiraled downward. She had two black eyes, swollen, purple lips, and an overly thin body covered with bruises that, to be truthful, made her look like one of the zombies from the latest horror movies.

She knew enough about her body to know that real damage had been committed, which later proved to be true when the doctors announced that having children would be questionable. She had always believed that it was important to have sex with someone you loved and respected with the reverse being true, as well, for she wanted to be respected, too. But she had given that all up when she had fallen in love with drugs and those powerful, wonderful feelings they gave her. In fact, she found that her body now joined with her mind in insisting on getting that drug feed each day. God! What was she going to do?

The police wanted information regarding the rape which she refused to give them. She wouldn't give those jerks anything! She knew enough about what happened to girls who turned in their boyfriends for abusing them. It never stopped and the police could do nothing about it. All you had to do is pick up any newspaper and read it for yourself to know how that worked. It was always the girl's fault.

Were those boys *really* to blame anyway? Hadn't it all been *her* fault that led her here? Who would believe her side of the story anyway? If only she could think straight. She would just have to try to figure it all out later. Right now, she needed sleep and plenty of it. She hoped that the shot the doctors had given her would help. What she really needed was a fix. God! She hoped this was just a bad nightmare and it would be over soon!

Because of the extent of her injuries and being under the age of 21, her parents had to be notified because this incident was related to a criminal act. She was frantic at the thought that her parents would find her this way. As she felt shame wash over her, all she wanted to do was die. How was she going to be able to straighten everything out? What was the point anyway?

She was becoming sick to her stomach and asked for a bed pan. The "fun" drugs were wearing off. Even with the painkiller drugs the doctors had given her, the pain was so great, she began to shake uncontrollably.

Vague memories filled her mind and what she could remember only brought more shame and disgrace to her. She was humiliated to be here!

The hospital wanted her to sign up for the rehab program at the hospital but the only problem was that in this state you needed to be over 21 to be considered for their particular program, which meant that her parents needed to sign her in. How could she possibly endure letting them know how she had wasted so many months at school at their expense? Further, at the beginning of the week, the school counselor warned her that her scholarship was in jeopardy. She couldn't even think about that now. What next?

She was so angry and sad, and felt that there was no hope that anything positive could come out of this. Thoughts flittered through her mind that maybe an overload of pills would end all of her pain and disgrace, once and for all. For truly, what were her options? She had hurt her parents in so many ways by being unreasonable in every discussion where they had questioned what was really going on with her. She had spent an enormous amount of their money on schooling which had no real positive results. She had lied about attending classes as some mornings she just couldn't get out of bed. She had even spent the money that was to pay for her way home for the holidays!

She knew the reality. She had become addicted to drugs; she was a liar and a cheat; she shirked her responsibilities and so much more – none good. Now, she had put herself in a position where having children was not likely. She had even put herself in debt with the supplier of the drugs she had come to need on a daily basis – no longer wanting them but needing them, nevertheless.

How was it possible for her to explain all of this? How could this ever be resolved? Would her parents disown her? They had put their foot down the last time they all were together that they were no longer willing to "waste" their money on poor grades. What was she going to do? How was she going to end all of this mess? She was beginning to think that there was no way out . . .

SCENARIO 2

Now let's look at a 45 year-old man who has a high profile position at a new technology company that has taken off like crazy with a new product that helps companies track their on-road employees' activities. He was the kind of guy that went to work early and left late because he became so focused on developing leading edge products that it was hard for him to leave at a reasonable hour. He was very competitive in that arena.

For years, research and development had been his number one priority and challenge. The rest of business had no allure for him. Only after having finally reached success in his early thirties, did he feel he could even begin to socialize with a few friends, in spite of his feeling awkward and not really at ease doing it. However, he ended up meeting the love of his life at 33, married her and today they have 3 children, two boys ages ten and eight and a daughter that just turned three.

Seven years ago, he became Senior Vice President in the company he had created with his partner developing technology products. Five years ago, he began to rely on his younger management team to take on the greater load of responsibilities so that he could spend more time with his family.

That had lasted for just about a year when his partner became ill with cancer, and he was forced to take on an even greater role with the company. That meant that it was left to him to be the main one to network with prospective clients for all their products, and with financial prospects for backing the R & D of new products that they wanted to develop. That had always been his partner's role. Now, there wasn't anyone else in the company who could do it on the level that the prospective clients demanded. He was uncomfortable socializing but soon learned the trick of downing a drink or two to relax him before he met with them and others he was now responsible to meet.

At first, he could take it or leave it, although a drink did seem to help him be a bit more witty and relaxed. But the more he had to socialize, the more he became dependent on that drink beforehand.

There was a nice enough bar just around the corner from work where it was easy enough to slip in and grab a drink before a meeting. Sometimes, he would be able to stay for an hour sipping his drink and playing a few games on one of the slot machines that the bar had just installed for the pleasure of their customers. It was fun to play and he never lost much more than $50 to $100 dollars. Sometimes, he won that amount, so what the heck? Nothing ventured, nothing gained.

He was beginning to feel greater and greater pressure from his wife to be home more often because she was feeling overwhelmed with all that it took to care for their three children. She tried not to nag him and be a good sport, but he knew her well enough to know that she meant what she said. She needed him home.

He felt guilty for having scheduled evening meetings at a time that allowed him his "relaxation" time and so he tried to schedule any evening meeting early enough that he would still be home in time to put the kids to bed. But that wasn't easy because much of the timing depended on the prospective customer's timeframe which often meant dinner meetings. He began to fix himself a cocktail or two before dinner those nights he did make it home in time.

His weekends were beginning to get crazy with all of his commitments to play golf nearly every Saturday, which was good for business. Plus, he liked to play and end up at the 19th hole with the others regurgitating all the shots they had made and missed. Golf was slowly beginning to encroach on some of their Sundays as well which wasn't pleasing his wife. God! How did people do it? Grow their business and keep peace at home? He was beginning to feel pressure all around!

Both he and his wife, like most of their friends, were excited to attend the opening of the new casino in town. It meant having spectacular shows to attend where they could see some of their favorite entertainers, new gourmet restaurants available where they could dine or just being able to have fun playing the penny slot machines or sometimes even playing poker at the tables.

In the beginning, he and his wife made a "date" night every Saturday and always ended up at the casino because that is where most of the fun was to be had. His wife loved going to the shows (there were so many to choose from) and both of them appreciated the excellent food from the highly touted restaurants there.

But soon the newness wore off and things slipped back into the old pattern of being so busy with the kids for her and business for him that those "date nights" soon became rare. Furthermore, his wife hated to see so much money spent on food and gambling which seemed to her to be just throwing money away. She was very good at budgeting and handling the household expenses, so she put her foot down. No more Casino!

She repeatedly noticed that her husband seemed to gulp down more than just one drink before dinner, something she had brought up to him a few days ago, which had only served to anger him. And that wasn't the first time she had said something about it either. Each time, he told her that what did she expect with so much pressure on him to produce at work and then come home to hear her complain? That was the last thing he needed; didn't she understand that?

He shouted that he didn't want to hear what she had to say because he didn't criticize her, did he? Why did she pick on him when he had enough on his mind? After all, he did more than his share to pay all the bills, didn't he?

Meanwhile, he became intrigued with the idea of mathematically figuring out his odds in the various poker games, trying to outwit the house. No one was going to tell him what he could or could not do. More and more, he found ways to try out his theories always with the positive thought that he and he alone would be able to find a way for he had a creative mind, didn't he?

He made up excuses that kept him away from home and the office and sneaked into the Casino where he felt relaxed with a drink or two at the poker table. He was sure no one would catch on to how he was playing his cards trying out his different methods. He had so much fun until he lost. Then he was taken over by the fear and shock of how much he had lost, which meant that he was forced to stay and continue playing until he could make up his losses. And most times that did not happen.

He continued to lie to his wife and his employees as to his whereabouts at times. That didn't make him feel good at all, but he couldn't tell them what he was up to. He would be mortified if they found out. And besides, he would get his money back and no one would know the difference, right?

He became angry. There came a surge in him to not let the house get the better of him, so a silent war began between him and the Casino. He was determined to get back every cent he had lost over the past few months. All those times he had fooled everyone at home when he had played only nine holes of golf so that he could get to the Casino only to lose! He didn't dare tell his wife that he had taken money out of their now dwindling savings account. What was he thinking? What had he done? He had to get it back!

He knew he drank too much and became aware that his hands began to shake at the end of the day until he got a drink into his system. Things were not good but he didn't know what to do about it. The other night he had raised his voice to the boys and they ducked behind the stuffed chair as if they thought he would hit them. He had had to turn around and walk away so they wouldn't see the anguish on his face as he swallowed his tears. My God! What kind of a monster was he turning into? His own children afraid of him? What was happening to him?

His wife had tried to talk to him about his drinking that night and afterward he couldn't control his anger and had ranted and raved so much so that she had turned her back to him in bed that night. That was something that the two of them had vowed never to do – never to go to bed angry! They had agreed that together they would always be able to work things out. Yet, this was happening more and more. What was going to happen to them as a couple? How much longer was she going to put up with him? He loved her. What would he do without her and the kids?

His business partner was in remission from cancer and was returning to work next month which would be a big relief for him. He discovered only yesterday that while he had been spending so much time away from work, he was on the tip of losing their largest account and he didn't think that he could save it. He better call in his partner for this. Yet, how was he going to explain the situation to his partner who had counted on him to handle everything? How could he tell his partner that he had let him down? Maybe he should just walk away from everything. His business would probably be better off without him and what about his family? They probably would be happier without him too!

He closed and locked the door to his office, sat down at his desk, rested his head in his hands and cried deep sobbing cries. What had happened to him? How had he gotten to where he was now? What was he going to do?

*****

If you were able to step into the shoes of the young lady and the middle-aged man and get just a glimpse of what it feels like to be spiraling downward because of choices made while fulfilling the needs of an ever demanding addiction, you know how powerful that addiction can be. You know in your heart that they both are good people simply making poor choices.

Take time to think about them. If you were the young lady or the middle-aged man, what would you do next? What choices would you make? Would you be able to turn your life around?

Then, put yourself in the shoes of the parents of the young lady or the wife and partner of the middle-aged man. What would you do? How would you handle these situations? Would you ever be able to trust your loved one again?

It is always easier to make decisions and choices for others, isn't it?

When you look at these kinds of situations or any real-life ones, it is so easy to find blame and to judge others or to think that someone deserves to be in the situation they are in. Yet, it is interesting to note some of the major common emotions that set each of them on their path to make the choices they did and to end up in the situations they were in. For each of them was failing at fulfilling other people's expectations of them; each was not able to love and accept him or herself; each continued to create more and more stress in their life with their poor choices; each created increased isolation with their secrets and ways of living their daily life; each was creating a spiral downward with sad consequences.

How do you go from having a few drinks to become a drunk? Or go from smoking pot to snorting coke? Or go from playing a penny slot machine to betting big at the tables?

Jay is representing addiction as an accumulation of choices. This can assist in understanding how the gunk accumulates and how each time it becomes more difficult to make a different choice and easier to make the same one. Every single time makes a difference. He is saying if they can say NO just once they have started the change.

Each time that someone who is addicted refuses to feed their addiction, does that denial accumulate?

Yes, it does. You can always build on that.

SOMETIMES I THINK THAT NO ONE SHOULD HAVE TO ENDURE ADDICTION

*Even if you think that no one should have to go through that, they must go through it because they **created** it. And by going through it they re-create it and move **through** it.*

SO IF YOU CREATE IT, YOU HAVE TO DO IT AGAIN?

Yes. There are ways that you can process on the other side and you don't have to come back into a lifetime to address these issues; it is just faster to do it in the same form that created the issues. To eventually get it right.

WHAT IF SOMEONE FEELS THEY HAVE TO CREATE A DIFFERENT PERSONA?

For those who feel more creative when using drugs, they are afraid to stop using drugs because they don't want to lose their creativity. They believe their power to create is triggered by the drugs, not realizing it is the drugs that have triggered the connection to the soul which is the power to create, and there are other ways to trigger the connection to the soul.

Look at the act of W.C. Fields — he was convinced that his comedy was only let loose when he was drinking. So he became what he portrayed and he fell into the trap of thinking that he did not have that ability within himself believing that it was the drug of choice - the alcohol — that was doing it, not realizing that he had tapped into his own creativity power accidently, through the use of alcohol.

FOR PEOPLE WHO LIVE WITH ADDICTS, WHAT IS A POSITIVE THING FOR THEM TO DO?

First and foremost, when you are living with anyone who has any kind of addiction that is extreme like what you are talking about here, not the obsessive compulsive behaviors, but the destructive behaviors — when you are living with or near someone like that, it is absolutely essential that you create your own balance — the only way to do that is through the spiritual journey. I cannot give anyone a recipe through the physical, mental, and emotional that will ensure their success. I can tell each and every one of you who are suffering through this, that if you will look to your own spiritual strength and your own love, you will be fine and everything that you do to raise yourself up will make a huge difference to the one that is in the addiction.

WHY? BECAUSE THEY ARE MODELING THE RIGHT WAY AND THE POSITIVE ENERGY?

They have that example of living as a model, but they also have that feeding of the deeper level of energy. Jay just said that "When I am lifted up, I lift up all men with me." The same thing happens with individuals who are living with addicts — any addicts of any sort. If the individuals living with them can lift their own vibrational frequencies up to a certain point, it's an automatic rising for the other one as well. So first and foremost, the most important thing to do when you love someone who is addicted is to learn to love yourself.

WHAT IS ONE OF THE HARDEST THINGS TO LEARN FOR SOMEONE COMING OUT OF ADDICTION?

Is to love themselves and they can only love others to the degree that they love themselves.

We are bombarded with mixed messages leaving us with not feeling confident or good about many of the past choices we have made for even simple things. There are so many choices in our life that it can be difficult to find a clear, single way of living or one that we won't stray from. And yet, that is point of living the human experience — free will, free choice.

So I asked Jay:

HOW DID YOU LET GO OF THE FEAR? HOW DID YOU LET GO OF THAT FEAR OF ATTACK BY THE CATS IN THAT LIFETIME YOU SHARED WITH US?

I didn't. That fear became a part of other fear. He says that lifetime he showed is also a result of fear. It is just the first time it came to the point of dominating his life and got his attention 24/7. He says that situation would not have been able to occur if I had not already fallen into fear about some other things other lifetimes. It was just that was the best example of it because that is when it became cemented and most people don't clear their fears.

SO YOU CAN LIVE IN THE HIGHER MIND AND LIVE SPIRITUALLY EVEN HAVING THOSE FEARS?

Yes. He did overcome some of them. He had some lifetimes where he made some good progress. He is not saying that it is still 100% that. But if you look at the thousands of lifetimes we have, there is fear in every lifetime. We clear some and we bring on a little bit more; it shifts its focus, its shape, whatever you want to call it, but yeah, he hadn't cleared it or he wouldn't have been trying to escape life.

WE ALL HAVE SOME FEAR IN US, DON'T WE?

Yes, we do. Everyone comes in with fears. There is no one on the planet who doesn't have fears that they are going to be dealing with. One of the key problems we have right now is the frenetic life style pretty much everywhere in the world, but especially here in the western culture. Individuals are taught to be on alert and to worry all the time so the feeling of homo stasis or the state of homo stasis, the feelings of peace, calm and all of this stuff are literally conditioned out of children from the time they are babies.

That needs to turn around to the point where the children who are coming in now have this as a genetic pattern. Soon we will be reaching the point that if we don't turn it around, it will be that the children coming in automatically are no longer peaceful in a state of homo stasis — there is going to be more and more of what we think of as the "problem" children. So that needs to change fairly fast or otherwise addiction is just going to soar!

Remember, feeling nervous, anxious and unsafe is the foundation of all fears which, of course, makes it the foundation of all addictions. And we only feel nervous, unsafe and so forth because we have that feeling of separateness.

AND WE ARE LOOKING OUTSIDE OF SELF FOR OUR IDENTITY, AS WELL?

Exactly. And isn't that weird? We feel completely separate and yet we look to those things that we feel are separate from ourselves to feel good about ourselves!

THANK YOU. LOVE YOU.

Love you, too.

Where there is love, there is healing.

CHAPTER 7

WHAT DO I HAVE TO DO TO LIVE WITHOUT ADDICTION NOW?

As you have read through this book, we venture to say that you have a greater understanding of addiction in general – what it is and how it works – and, in particular, some of Jay's addictions highlighted in a few of his lifetimes. You also had a look at the experiences of two other individuals who got caught up in their addiction only to leave them wondering whether it was worth it for them to continue to live or not.

You have had the opportunity to appreciate from a spiritual sense how our individual energies are a culmination of our experiences that ultimately are tied to our state of being in reference to our connection to Source (God). In sharing this information, we have said that you will find joy, peace, love and happiness if you just do what we say. But that is not total reality because we are individual and live on different levels of spiritual growth, that which acknowledges that we all are one.

Yet, the reality is that all of us, each one, have the same goals in life whether recognized or not. For who doesn't want all the best things in life? For those with addictions, we want to be free of them. We all want to be loved and loving; live without fear; love, accept and forgive ourselves for actions taken that are not to our highest good or the highest good of others; want to be successful (whatever that is for each of us), and want to have joy and happiness in our life, along with good health.

But before we look into the different ways of higher mind living, we need to look again at what makes an addict move into the space of wanting and seeking help to recover.

First of all, you have to have that "spark" of something that gets you from where you are in a place of discomfort to "Boy, I am sick of my life, and I know that there has to be something better - a better life for me." That "spark" that lets you know it's true.

SO JAY, CAN YOU SHARE EITHER WORDS OF WISDOM OR CAN YOU EXPLAIN HOW THOSE MANY TIMES YOU WENT INTO REHAB YOU WENT FROM HITTING BOTTOM TO SEEKING HELP?

When you called it that "spark of life" that is exactly what it is. It is that moment when you reach complete desperation and desolation. That is the moment where we are either the most open to salvation from our higher self or soul and also the most closed depending on the individual. It is also the moment when we have the most dynamic assistance beamed into our energy.

When I was at that moment, I had a lot of help. It wasn't just from the other side- it was the thought of my mother. It was the thought of what would happen to her, and because there was that bond between the two of us, it was like an additional crow bar being used to pry open the door to the light and, of course, I had a lot of help from the other side as well. But it became an issue of where is my greatest fear. Is my greatest fear of life or death? And it boils down to that for a lot of people.

Many of the ones who deliberately commit suicide are more afraid of life than death as they think of it because, of course, there is no such thing as not being. But there is kind of like an overview of all your beliefs, your hopes and fears in a split second. In that moment, you decide if you are attached to fear or hope. If you are attached to fear or power, power is a better way of putting it. Those who are lucky enough to have someone who truly loves them and they love them in return have a much better chance of coming up on the beam of power rather than to continue going down on the beam of fear. And it is actually a very simple yet complicated process. It is a simple matter of choice, but the complication comes in on the split second timing of each individual's openness to redemption, salvation, hope, power or whatever you want to call it. In my case, a lot of it was flavored by the memories of when times were better.

Like you had said earlier, there were times when I was in rehab I had hope; I had strength, and I could remember those. I had times when I was on the brink, and you came in and helped me come back in off the brink. I had experiences that aimed me in the direction of power instead of fear.

What is that spark of change that builds the bridge from hitting bottom to connecting to source?

It has to do with the experiences here in the lifetime. I had those experiences in rehab because when I was in there I had the feelings of power, hope, strength and all the good stuff. The problem is it is a million times easier to stay free of a bad habit when you are in a controlled environment like where you are told exactly what to do and how to do it, and you are given guarantees that it will work as long as you do this, and you have no choice but to do that anyways!

In those times when I was in rehab, I had proof that I could beat it; proof that it was possible. But then when I came out of that environment, that very, very, controlled environment, and went back into the environment of choice, and went back into the environment of that hodge-podge of what is presented to me, it was the hodge-podge slowly wearing me down – a little bit here, a lot there – that would take me right down to the bottom again. It's like coming up with a challenge while in the spirit vs. coming up with a challenge while in the physical. The controlled environment of rehab is like coming up with a challenge in spirit. Real life is coming up with a challenge in life, a challenge in the physical.

But I had the experiences in that lifetime of feeling my own power and that made a huge difference. It doesn't for everyone because not everyone who goes into rehab feels that. A lot of them don't want to be there and they fight it. I DID want to be there.

Past lives come into it as well. How many times have we made the choice of power over fear? And how many times have we made the choice of fear over power?

SO IF I AM ADDICTED AND WANT TO GET BETTER AND I HAVE THAT SPARK OF SOMETHING BUT DON'T KNOW WHERE TO BEGIN, WHAT IS THE FIRST THING I SHOULD DO?

Cut yourself off from anyone or anything that is a bridge to that addiction. If you have a best friend that you smoked pot with, cut yourself off from him.

SHOULD I GO TO THE HOSPITAL IF I DON'T KNOW WHO TO TURN TO?

Depends on each individual — each will respond differently. He should seek professional help any way he can, which will take a lot of humbling because most people who are addicted don't want to admit they are because they feel it is a weakness, it is something someone is going to take away from them, etc. etc. So humility is extremely important. Not the humility that says I am a piece of crap, but the humility that says you know that I need some help.

Humility is difficult for people with addictive behaviors. When you have an addictive behavior, what you are really doing is escaping from what you perceived is the reality of your life which says your life isn't good enough, which means you are not good enough, the people around you aren't good enough - however you want to look at it

WE KNOW THAT FEAR IS AT THE SEAT OF ADDICTION AND WE KNOW THAT LOTS OF TIMES WE CARRY FORWARD THAT FEAR. AND IF WE WANT TO GO BACK TO THOSE LIFETIMES AND CONFRONT IT SO THAT WE CAN CLEAR IT, WE UNDERSTAND IT HAS TO DO WITH FEELINGS. IF WE CAN ACCEPT THOSE FEELINGS CAN WE CLEAR THE FEAR AND LET GO OF THE FEAR?

There is a difference between accepting feelings and acknowledging them. If we do it the way we want to, we simply acknowledge the feelings, but we do not accept their reality because they are fear-based. We accept the reality that we have created them, that we are living in them, but we do not accept the reality in the sense of power. We do not accept them as a part of who we are. We simply acknowledge their presence – oops, we made a boo-boo. We created this thing and we give it absolutely no power by acknowledging that it is simply something we created that we are not going to re-create. There are many who do not want to accept the kind of power we are talking about here. Remember every individual is going to respond differently. So we are giving some general terms but that is all they are – they are just general understanding because every individual is different because of their experiences.

But in this case, you would look at it as acknowledging the existence of what you might call a weakness or an addiction is different for everyone too. One person might acknowledge it and say "Oh yeah. I am an addict and I get what I want out of it and I feel damn good; I feel powerful; I feel in control, and I'm keeping it!" Another person might look at it and say, "Well, there is nothing I can do about it. Poor me. I just have to keep this." Another might look at it as your son Jay did and say "I just have to keep fighting it." All three of these are the most common reactions, but they are not the most desired reactions.

Even "I have to keep fighting it" gives the addiction more power than it should have because we only fight things that have power over us. So when you say accepting that a condition exists, accepting is a good word in the sense that we have created it and acknowledged it, but many of them accept it as WHO they are and they use it either as an excuse to continue the same way, as an excuse to not do anything – that sort of thing. And it is important for people to start learning the difference.

Anytime we need anything to give us a shift in our emotional and mental focus, there is the potential of addiction. There is a level of addiction (in our jargon we wouldn't call it an addiction at all (more like a hankering) but it does plant a seed for that potential. And we all do it, every single one of us, whether we have a ritual of a glass of wine in the evening or something else. We all have something we use.

WHEN YOU TALK ABOUT THAT YOU FELT POWERFUL, IN WHAT WAY?

I felt powerful in the way to overcome the addiction. I was given step-by-step formulas and a guarantee that if you do this, you can come out of it. And I was given proof of it because while I was in rehab, I started feeling better, stronger and, therefore, more in control of my life, which we think of as being powerful. And I had an experience of that in the mental, emotional and physical body because of my reaction to rehab, and it made a huge difference for me. It was just when I got out of the controlled environment that I didn't have the structure to lean on anymore, and I didn't have the strength to create it for myself even though I had a loved one who would have gladly created it for me. The problem is that you couldn't wrap me in cotton and stick me in a room. And that is about what it would have taken.

Jay says "Bottom line, I enjoyed being high too much. It was a complete escape."

I LOOK AT THAT RELATIONSHIP OF THE FEELING YOU GET FROM A HIGH FROM DRUGS, ALCOHOL, GAMBLING OR WHATEVER AS BEING IT IS WHAT IT IS AND CANNOT BE TRULY "REPLACED." CAN IT BE SET ASIDE?

They are saying that you can't really set it aside. They know what you are talking about in the sense of not being active with it and all that stuff, but what Jay is saying is that in rehab, they try to tell you to just put it over on a shelf and then go work on your spiritual or emotional stuff. They don't realize that all that energy involved in that high has to be incorporated into the search for spiritual living.

Jay says yes, you have to set it aside, put it out of your mind, you have to do this instead of that, but that is creating an exclusion. Life does not allow exclusions. Anything that is excluded will persist in trying to come in because it used to be part of the whole. And anything that is placed outside of love cannot be healed. As long as the rehab center says that you have to set it aside, it is not going to work.

Now Jay is talking about bringing that energy of the high, the kind of high they felt on the drug, remembering that feeling and incorporating that into the spiritual quest. Once the body, mind and emotions experience the high like that, you can re-create it to a certain degree – re-creating it with control and purpose so it is not dangerous anymore, it is not drug induced, and all of that. Shifting the vibrational frequencies helps take out the addictive quality from that feeling of high and putting in the spiritual quality.

[Regina Murphy, a pioneer of sound therapy has created tools that do this. You can go to www.soundsforselftreatment.com to find many healing tools.]

If people only realized that once they experience that drug addiction, you hook yourself – if you do it once, you have the seed of addiction right there. But once you have experienced it in order to make gold out of "poop," you can go into your body, mind and emotions and allow those feelings of bliss to be re-created in a natural way. It won't be off the charts and out of control like it is with the drugs – thank goodness – yet, it will be the body, mind and emotions way of remembering feeling the lightness. But it has to be done in the sense of incorporating in love, not that I want this feeling to get away from life.

SO I CAN TAKE THE FEELING HIGH FROM SEXUAL INTERCOURSE OR DRUGS OR ALCOHOL OR ANY ADDICTION AND BRING THAT FEELING TO MIND AS I WATCH A BIRD BUILD A NEST OR SIMPLY WASH MY HANDS AND SO FORTH?

Yes. You become more aware of what is around you, and instead of escaping from life, you are using those feelings for appreciation for and connection with life. So we incorporate that high with life, but at the same time, it is extremely important to adjust the frequencies of what you are incorporating so you don't get that negative aspect of it because that is all about escaping life. Drugs are all about escaping life, and you don't want that.

SO YOU TAKE HOW YOU FELT ON DRUGS AND REPLACE THOSE GOOD FEELINGS (ELIMINATING THE NEGATIVE ONES) WITH THE HIGHER WAY OF LIVING AND THE CONNECTION TO SOURCE?

Yes, and incorporate that with living life in the physical body. The biggest problem people run into here is that the drugs are an instant fix.

WELL, THE HIGHS CAN ALMOST BE INSTANT TOO, THE REGULAR HIGHS WHEN YOU DEVELOP IT TO THAT POINT, RIGHT?

Yes, it just takes time and patience to develop it and some determination, of course.

IT ALSO COMES ABOUT WITH THE REALIZATION THAT NOTHING STAYS HIGH ALL THE TIME.

That's right. It's not realistic. You have hit a very important point. It does take persistence and determination and consistency. There is no such thing as a magic wand.

That's why so many are getting upset with things like The Secret. That was such an important major step but people thought it was everything. They showed the highs all the time just like you said and people said "Oh good, I will start thinking like that and I will have the high all the time" and it doesn't work that way. It's a piece of the puzzle, just not the whole thing.

We had discussions with Jay for some of the best ways to get into a higher state of mind, the higher frequencies, that would make life more powerful for us in a spiritual sense. By doing so, we would be less apt to opt out of life by using our addictions for escape. It is interesting to note that in order for us to live *without* addiction *now*, we simply are setting the same intentions and goals that we would to create all the best things in life - a double whammy for bringing in peace, joy, and love of All That Is!

One of our strongest instincts is survival, that desire for continued existence. We know that after using drugs and alcohol for an extended period of time that need to survive can be diminished because of an altered state of being, physically, mentally, and spiritually. We can begin to become blind to the joy of living and start to feed our sense of "less than" with any of that feel good euphoria that comes from choosing whatever it is we are using to get us into that higher state of being. How do we get back to that place of good health in both body and mind? Is it possible? How do we get from the entrapment of addiction to a space of wanting to be addiction free to being able to be spiritually, physically and mentally free of addiction?

Jay says that miracles are alive and well in the 21st century and explained that many of those miracles for addicts come by way of a sudden thought that life is more than what the addict is living, and his or her belief that they can have and deserve that better life. Miracles are more than serendipity. They are gifts from God, available to all of us, often coming to us through a connection to others, even strangers. Life comes alive when you become *aware* of all around you which opens yourself up to receiving all miracles, small and large. You begin to look around and see so much that identifies all the ways that we are connected to each other and to God (our Source).

What happens then is that we begin to find an inner peace because we now understand that *we* are the creators of our life, and *we* have the power to change our life by what *we* think, say and do.

Before we can create our success in shattering the power of addiction and living without addiction now, we need to understand our role in accomplishing this. Having an addiction to anything is something we all deal with in some form or another. By providing you in simple terms some of the most concrete ways that are available in today's society to release addiction, along with other ways to raise your vibration to a higher mind existence, we do not mean to sound glib. It is not something you wake up and do/be and then the next day everything is fine and you no longer have addictions.

Again, what these methods really do is awaken you to ways that bring you to a state of living in the NOW so that you are no longer worrying about where your next "fix" is coming from. Living in the now means that you are in that state of accepting that all is as it should be, and when it isn't, *you* have the power to create something better. It is a knowing peace within that if you do your best to live a life full of love with the capability to both give and receive love, life flows with goodness. It is an ever increasing awareness of the beauty that surrounds you filling you with gratitude for being able to experience it. It is a connection with Source that allows you to know and be love in ways not yet experienced. It is a fulfillment of the light of All That Is.

Can you live WITHOUT ADDICTION NOW? Absolutely!

How? As you know, when you change your addiction from a lower mind to a higher mind, you are actually changing thought patterns from the conscious mind to the subconscious mind where the higher intelligence (Universe) exists.

One of the suggested ways is hypnosis but only with a professional that is experienced, preferably one in dealing with addiction. During hypnosis or self-hypnosis you can actually **instruct** your subconscious mind. For example, you might say, "I am instructing you to find opportunities to bring more peace into my life and find ways to do it without drugs (or whatever your addiction is). Say it, and leave it up to the subconscious to find the ways because the subconscious will work at it until it finds some of those ways that will work. *However, this is important to remember, you need to have the lower mind (individual mind that is stuck in survival) agree with the higher mind (connection to Source) in order for addiction to cease.* And this for most of us takes time and building steps to create that agreement because the lower mind where addiction lives wants to be boss. Because our earth is raising its vibration, going into the higher dimensions, that timetable is becoming less and is more and more doable in a shorter amount of time, depending upon where you are in your mind – your state of being.

THIS IS KEY: Let's look again at "agreement." You cannot have a belief unless you AGREE to it. For instance, if you are told that you are stupid enough times, you begin to believe it because slowly you have become in agreement with it whether you are aware of it or not. When you realize that you are not stupid, that is not because you didn't BELIEVE it a one time, it is because you no longer AGREE with it. And that is how it can be with addiction. You can suddenly have a moment when you no longer AGREE with being an addict or even more so, you no longer AGREE that you need to pick up that drink, drug or do anything tied to your addiction because continued addiction does not AGREE with your higher power (mind) and WHO you are.

We want to *clear* our addictions and don't want to be beholden to owning it forever even if we believe we have it "under control." Let's be specific, having addiction "under control" is not the same thing as *clearing* it. We want to *clear* it so that we don't have to work through it again another lifetime. We want to re-establish that connection with God (Source) so that each lifetime, we have memory of how to live our life all the ways that are best for us and for all.

You may not even be aware of an issue you are working on. Yet similar situations come back at you again and again, sticking to you like gum to a shoe! This is you and the Universe working together to create the opportunity to look at a similar situation again and give you the occasion to clear it. Always remember the Universe wants the best for us and will continue to provide with love another chance for you to experience and clear a situation within a lifetime. However, I must be clear. You do not get back the *same* experience to clear now or in another lifetime although you can choose the same issue to work on and clear, such as alcoholism.

Each one of us has our own journey with so many aspects to it that there is no magic wand that will put everyone quickly and easily on a path where there are no addictions UNLESS you do your part. But we can promise you that, if you use some of the ways below and even research them in greater detail via the computer or books read or classes taken, your life will be different. Some of these methods take time and repetition to bring you to the state of mind that you want and deserve. Although the journey of self-growth is not always easy, it is glorious! And trust us. It is worth your effort in a positive way not only for you, but for all those around you.

When using some of the methods listed below to become a greater higher-mind being, you will see that it all boils down to energy. Everything is ENERGY, every single thing.

How does this work? Every thought you have has energy, and when you speak those thoughts, the energy becomes even greater with the action being the result of the thought, the word or both. It is interesting to note that words have more power now than in any other time since that of Jesus! So heed the warning to take care what words you speak and what thoughts you have for it no longer takes much time for the Universe to respond to your thoughts or words or actions. The vibrational energy is that powerful.

Also, as our earth and your own vibrations become higher, the response from the Universe is almost immediate, making it easier and quicker for you to manifest what you want. Remember, oftentimes, when we ask the Universe for something and we don't receive it, there is something better coming to us. Always ask the Universe for what you want and add "or something better." In other words, *don't limit* the Universe to what it can give you. Ask the Universe in such a way that there is no confusion as to what it is you are requesting because the Universe isn't able to guess what you want. You can even use the words, "I command . . . "(whatever it is you want).

Before we go onto the list of actions that we can do to help us live without addiction, we need to understand the **Law of Attraction.** It simply states that what you give out energetically is what is returned to you, and what you focus on is what you create. I like to use the visual of the toy paddle board with a ball tied to it with a long rubber band. Each time you hit the ball with the paddle, the ball returns. Think of yourself as the paddle, what you think, say or do as the ball, and the rubber band as the Universe. You get the picture, right?

So each time you send out love, it is returned to you, sometimes in loving ways you never thought possible. And the same thing happens when you send out angry words, judgments, or anything negative. It is not so much fun to be on the receiving end of that, for sure, as negativity is like a cancer that spreads easily without regard for anyone in the way. It also takes longer to heal from negativity. You can easily create the persona you want by your thoughts, words and actions, and that is part of your power.

Now, the important thing to know is that *your* energy affects the whole. You are part of the mass consciousness. A very simple example would be if you started your day grumpy, angry and unhappy. Later, when you are with other people, your negative energy may still be around you, and suddenly those others around you may pick up your negative energy and they, in turn, may also become grumpy, etc. Keep in mind, like energies support each other.

Yet, the opposite is true. Think of the times you have walked down the street and smiled at others and they returned the smile. That joy energy (simply a higher energy) is infectious. Remember Jay's lifetime where he stumbled into the man with the high energy and the effect it had on him? The bottom line is that what you think, say and do creates your choices and the good or bad in your life.

So it is important to follow the methods of high-mind living listed below and create the life of your dreams! You can do it!

An **Affirmation** is a powerful, positive statement about something you would like to have happen has already happened. This helps the mind and subconscious believe it is reality, and that belief needs to be in place before you can manifest it to be so. If you say the words, and your subconscious mind does not believe it can be so, it won't happen.

For instance, how many people would like to be wealthy but are not because deep down inside they don't believe they *deserve* to be? Or they believe they have to *earn* it.

Jays says *as soon as you have to earn something, you can't really have it. If you have to earn it, you have to chase it. If you live in the space of having to earn it, you never deserve it. You can never have what you don't deserve. In truth you deserve everything, but if you put yourself in a mental and emotional position of not deserving, that is the reality you create for yourself – you can't have it. It's about allowing.*

Sometimes, even if you think your affirmation seems silly or may never happen, all you need to do is begin saying a few affirmations building upon the belief that you can have it. Each time you put yourself into the energy of affirming what you want, the reality of that becomes greater because without being aware of it, you create the space to *allow* it to happen and believe it to be so.

However, when you state affirmations, they are encoded with your mood. So in order for affirmations to work, you must state them not thinking in terms of moving AWAY from anything – rather as MOVING TOWARD what you want. You need to be in the right state of mind of expectancy that what you are asking for is going to happen.

The two most creative words are I AM. As soon as you say I AM anything, it is in the now – it already exists. Again, because words are so powerful, it is important to be aware of the words we use, especially in light of using I AM affirmations. It is essential to use positive words only. Why would you want to use negative words anyway? I AM is the God self and the most powerful two words we can use.

Simple affirmations such as, I am happy, I am healthy, or I am anything can easily be expanded so the Universe knows how to better provide for you. For instance, express all the ways that you are happy. Remember you are the only one who can make yourself happy. No one else can make you happy although they can provide situations that provide you happiness. So again, in your affirmation of "I am happy" express all the different ways that provides you happiness. Visualization helps with that, too.

Even making a vision board provides greater energy for the manifestation of what you desire. For instance, "I am happy" can become I am happy when I drive my new red sports car because it is safe for my family when we take a ride together. Now you can add more ... the car smells so new and fresh and is a happy smell to me; how it looks, feels and more. Hang a picture of the car on your vision board or whatever you want to create in your life and use affirmations to go along with it. Combining these things provides a greater energy for what you want to come to fruition. The Universe doesn't know any different than what you ask for and the energy surrounding it.

That type of affirmation is pretty simple for us to do because, for the most part, it removes us from our inner feelings that we have about our self. However, have you ever stood in front of a mirror and told yourself that you love you? Or that you are a beautiful person without listing all your "deficiencies?" It is so difficult for most of us to appreciate and love ourselves without a list of judgments against our own self, forgetting that we are much more critical of us than any other ten people combined would be!

It is very important for all of us to affirm with the Universe who we are remembering that the Universe loves us *no matter what*. We have to love and accept ourselves as perfect beings sometimes doing imperfect things and that we are all one. We are all in the same creative energy here on earth, and it is important to honor that. Forgive yourself for being human! Remember you can't love someone fully unless you love yourself.

Jay says, *accept, accept, accept!*

Another thing to help you in your desire to rid yourself of addictions is **Alcoholics Anonymous ["AA"] and Other Support Groups.**

A good reminder is what Jay says, *Life is about "unpiling"; about letting go; and about love.*

Earlier, Jay discussed ways to strengthen AA and support groups, but always with the understanding that it is very important for anyone with addictions to have the support of others as long as the support is positive and not defeatist. When you find that you are not in a "good place" with your addiction, it is important to surround yourself with those like-minded people whose energy can lift you up into a higher level of vibrational energy where you can cope more easily with whatever issue you are dealing with. Support groups can be very positive for there is strength in numbers that can remove you from a space of feeling all alone.

Like anything else, it is important to assess the group for yourself to make sure that the people in it are those that are determined to replace their addiction with other things in life that serve them better. And that they want to move on without allowing attending meetings to simply become another addiction. You don't want to be in a space of thinking that you can't do anything or go anywhere unless you attend a meeting. Meetings are intended to be supportive, not essential to survival; they are intended to encourage you to become strong on your own with your personal connection to God; they are there for support.

Your support group needs to be an environment where you can feel safe to say whatever you are feeling or to express ideas. It should be a place where roles within the group are shared and everyone is involved without judgment of each other or their experiences.

Your support group shouldn't keep you shackled as an addict; rather, as someone who *used to* have an addiction, someone who is addiction free.

What should you do if you haven't found the right group for you yet?

Try another! There are so many wonderful, beautiful people who will help you that you will soon find yourself in the perfect place before you know it.

A good reminder is that many times we are offered the opportunity to let others be "in service" to us and assist us in many ways. Yet, we often feel uncomfortable letting them do so. Those are the times that allow others to demonstrate their love energy which is so important for their spiritual growth. So don't be afraid to ask for help when you need it and *let them help you!*

Chakra work is another thing to help you clear your negative energies. There are seven major chakras (energy portals) of our body beginning at the bottom of our spine to just above the crown of our head. *Jay says at this point in development, it is a good idea to look at them as individualized streams of energy. It helps people work with them and it helps people sort out their own individual issues. After trauma, you need finite. Like with you and me.*

When we separate each one, we can tie that energy to different body parts and emotions. Each of the seven has it owns color representing it, and other things increase the energy of the chakras, such as the colors of different crystals, herbal oils, flowers, yoga positions, and much more. Jay reminds us that color is going to be a major healer of health issues, including addiction. When you have all of your seven major chakras in balance, there is a free flow of energy within your body which initiates the healing of all that needs to be healed.

Spiritually, we are given information all the time and when we ignore that information, we are given information mentally. If we ignore both of those avenues, the chakras physically let us know what is going on regarding both physical and emotional issues. I call chakras the "blabber mouths" of our system because they let us know if we have a blockage.

I asked Jay:

NOW WITH THIS FLOW OF ENERGY, HOW IS THAT GOING TO HELP ADDICTION?

Think of addiction as a mean octopus. It wraps it tentacles around you until you cannot move. It's a very locked and low energy. Now imagine that an energy comes in that is light and fluffy. It's like a cartoon – the energy starts to permeate that dark, low octopus and the octopus starts to become kind of "spongy" and "floaty" and begins to loosen its hold. It's a rather crude way of looking at it, but that is basically it. Addiction keeps you locked in the lower vibrations.

You have always been correct in cleaning up those lower chakras because it involves the love of self, which is the center for all. Sometimes, people cannot go straight into the heart and throat chakras. Sometimes, some garbage needs to be hauled out first. Now some of these that are addicted are addicted because they are searching for the feelings they had on the other side, and some are addicted because they are escaping the feelings they have on this side. You will find that as the vibrational frequency continues to increase, there will be a lot more pressure on the people with addictive personalities. There will be more clear choice, more turmoil for many of them because of the struggle because of the contrast between the two. The greater the contrast, the greater the struggle. So some of them are in the deepest holes while here and some of them will ascend. This is a time of miracles.

It will take a bit of time for you to understand and learn about the chakras, but it will be worth your effort. Chakra is a Sanskrit word meaning disc or wheel and represents a center of spiritual energy in the body, usually considered to be 7 in number as the major chakras. Just know, that by understanding the chakras, you will have greater power to create the life you want. There are many books available to you on the subject; in fact, you can go to www.amazon.com and look for the three books on chakras written by me – *The Seven Major Chakras, Keeping it Simple* and *A Simple Approach to Living a Successful Life* and *What You Need to Know to Live a Spiritual Life.*

Exercise is one of the *most effective quick releases of endorphins* (that feel good chemical produced by our body or falsely created by chemicals we put into our body).

Jay says physical movement is imperative for anyone who is in any kind of addiction. All addictions settle as energy within the physical body, and it affects the nerves, tendons, the neuron pathways in the body, and every aspect that is energy in the physical body. The physical body is energy so anytime that you are dealing with mental, emotional or physical addictions of any kind, physical movement can be a breakthrough. There must be a consistent approach to a healthy moving of the body on a regular basis every single day, and if individuals will allow themselves to do that, it can be key to making the process so much easier.

The issue with the addictions is that it takes away the drive to do anything of that nature, of a positive nature, where you are nurturing. So they are challenged with JDI (just do it). It literally comes to a point where if you are sitting on the couch, stand up and do the yoga stretches. Don't say, should I do it now, should I do it later, or I don't want to do it. Just stand up and do it! That is a lot of what is required in coming out of addictions. It is the determination to gain control of one's life or to regain one's life.

So first and foremost, the easiest way we can recommend to individuals is healthy movement of the body, the easiest and most immediate way. Of course, that alone will not take care of the issue, as you know. Bottom line - there is a break in spirituality when you venture into addictions. All addictions are based in fear; all fear is based in being alone and being in threat for non-survival. When we can once again come into the feeling of connectedness - that positive light either with other human beings, animals, friends on the other side (such as we who serve you here - God itself), then that addiction no longer holds power. So we give you physical as the easiest, fastest to begin with, but as we said before, the bottom line is the connection, the Oneness.

So in order to come out of addiction, anyone who is addicted in any way must seek themselves and who they really are in the sense of the Source and the

Oneness. Most of the individuals need to start with cleaning out the junk, cleaning out the negative emotions, the fear patterns, all of these things. There are many really fine modalities that are available on the earth plane at this time.

So first to jump start, you are going to do the physical exercise. It would be good if it is the kind of physical exercise you enjoy, but many in addiction don't enjoy anything but the addiction – so remember, just do it. Get off the couch, stand up and do it!

When you are walking or doing anything that is repetitive, that is the perfect time to let your mind float and connect with the higher mind. Remember, part of how you make that connection with the higher source is to become *aware* of everything around you, particularly all that Mother Earth provides us: plants, animals, the sky and its clouds, changes in weather, etc. and you will be able to see how it and we are all connected. You will be able to feel and sense a higher power because you will be in that space of knowing it is so.

When you finish with any kind of exercising, you should be on a higher energy plane that allows you to believe that you can do anything you set your mind to do because you have connected with Source. The more you work with the other methods to raise your vibration, and the more you combine it with exercise, the greater the chance of replacing addiction by simply living a satisfying life ... one without addiction.

Does that sound doable? It is. Try it!

If I AM are the two most creative words, **Gratitude** is one of the most productive emotions. When you are in a state of gratitude for all that is in your life and you state that with love, you are in the space of the highest vibrational frequency. Yet, this is such a simple thing to do that it may be difficult to understand just how powerful its effectiveness is.

Gratitude, simply put, is your recognition of a higher source (God) expressed in many forms. When you say thank you for whatever it is, you are acknowledging a blessing in your life, a realization that you have been given a gift whether it is an actual thing, idea or thought, an emotion of love or an experience to help you understand what you didn't before.

Gratitude expressed is an energy that fills you with the same energy that heals – the love energy. Don't be stingy with expressing all your appreciation to those around you, even inert objects, along with other living things, that aren't able to communicate with you, such as your dog, birds, and the like. Gratitude is powerful and is something to build on to bring joy of living into your life. When we grow the number of things that we are grateful for, it makes us aware of the connection to all in existence both on earth and on the other side. That connection becomes *everything* bringing us peace to be where we are in life surrounded by the unconditional love of the Oneness. It releases the stresses of living here on the planet.

Healthy Food is a must. We are so spoiled here in America for all the choices and amounts of food that are available to us, which makes it easy to consume unhealthy food, particularly since so much of our prepared food has unhealthy chemicals in it. It is important to look at how we are filling our bodies by what we are choosing to eat. The more that we get away from the natural foods coming from Mother Earth, the more we are susceptible to creating "dis-ease" within our bodies.

Jay says *that as we get into lighter and lighter bodies we won't need red meat. But there are those in physical bodies now that still need the enzymes available in red meat that you haven't figured out how to get anywhere else. So it isn't that they are bad, it is that their body recognizes the need. The problem is that they take in the chemicals at the same time and they take in the consciousness of the brutality of the way the beasts were raised.*

There have been programs on television that show places in Japan, and even a few in other countries, where slaughter houses recognize that soft music played for the animals and an orderly line up of those about to be slaughtered make a positive difference energetically. After all, why shouldn't they be honored for having given up their life in order to sustain ours?

Because most of us have no control over how the meat, vegetables, grains and fruit were treated on their route to us, we can still honor and change any negative energy into a more loving one by thanking each part of the food we ingest when we say our blessing before we eat. It makes a notable difference to have that changed energy within our digestive system.

Why is it important to get healthy? When we don't, we remain in the lower vibrational energies that bar us from becoming lighter in spirit, and good health. Although our bodies are just our "houses" here on the earth plane, they are to be honored and maintained so that we can live a healthy, happy life without the stress of poor health and illness.

Be Aware: We use so many chemicals and color enhancers in our food that it is literally making people and animals sick, and in some cases, causing death. One of the worst offenders is **SUGAR.** Yet, nearly all of us are ADDICTED to sugar in one form or another. Instead of eating things that are organic, our society is more concerned with how its products look and what price they can bring, willing to push aside what is best for us, and have its goal monetary gain. Have you noticed how many people around you are sick or have died from cancer? Have you wondered if it has anything to do with what they eat or have eaten? Maybe the water or other liquids ingested? How many people today are overweight, particularly children? What can YOU do? Learn what you are eating and what is best for you to eat to remain healthy. Read the labels of the foods you buy and choose those that are the healthiest for you.

Mediation is something that we should do every day.

*Jay says that **meditation** is the greatest way to strengthen the positive and connect with the higher vibrations — that lightness that we seek through addictions.*

It is not always easy to clear your mind of all the earthly ties, leaving behind thoughts of things to do, financial worries or anything negative that may be occurring in your life. But if you put on music that soothes your soul and sit with your body aligned, and face your palms to the sky to receive messages and energies from the Universe, you will begin to find inner peace. Breathing deeply, inhaling through your nose and exhaling out your mouth, releases old energy and brings in fresh oxygen and new energy that helps you relax and ready yourself for your meditation.

There are different types of meditation. There are learning meditations that will teach you new ideas, and if your meditation is on a CD, you can play it over and over until you are comfortable with it; there are music-only meditations where you can relax and quiet yourself to allow consciousness to go to nothingness; there are guided meditations where you are led different places with different thoughts; there are yoga-based meditations for you to position yourself in different ways; and, of course, there is meditation where you simply stop what you are doing no matter where you are and position yourself with closed eyes for your own escape.

"No matter how you choose to meditate, the results wished for are always the same. It boils down to giving yourself over to your higher power and simply letting things be. As you meditate and leave behind your worries, you will feel a connection to your higher mind, higher self, and higher power, understanding that all is as it should be. This gives you the strength to deal with life as it presents itself, acknowledging that you are here to experience all of life.

What you may discover by meditating is how to prioritize how you choose to live. For those of you who have travelled by airplane, you have heard the flight attendants state in their instructions to please drop down the oxygen mask and place it on you first before attending to another travelling with you who needs your help.

That may sound selfish to you at first until you realize that if you cannot breathe, you can't help anyone else. And that is the way it is in life. You have a responsibility to take care of yourself in all the best ways so you are in a position to help others. For that is what living a successful life is all about – a life without addiction and helping others when needed and is to everyone's best interest. Everything in your life begins and ends with you: the choices you make; the love you create and share; and the gratitude you express.

The quickest, easiest way to lift yourself up without drugs or any outside influences is through meditation. It is your opportunity to become one with all; your opportunity to connect with self; your opportunity to know unconditional love.

Jay says, Meditate, meditate, meditate!

Music. You may have heard the expression that "music is the language of the Gods" which indicates how we view the importance of music and sound. Music is a powerful tool which has the ability to stir up our emotions and the way we feel. It also has the power through its tones to heal. I encourage you to go to Regina Murphy's website *www. soundsforselftreatment.com*. Regina talks and shows how music shifts your frequency, which can actually change your DNA to help you heal!

Remember when Jay was talking about doing and being? If we listen to music with words, we are really still in a state of doing; if we listen to music without words, we can reach that state of being by letting ourselves go into a meditative state. In order to connect to our higher self and connect to source, it is important to be in that state of being for greater results.

Much of classical music is considered to be mathematical, which is why children are encouraged to listen to it when they are young. Without identifying why, classical music has the ability to soothe and calm and keep one focused on being. We believe that it ties us into the energy grids of the earth plane where our thoughts and remembrances all become clear and begin to make sense to us.

Sound is something each of us can create whether we sing or bang pots or beat on drums or anything else that produces sound. It is interesting to note that once you start making sound any way that you can, after a while you will automatically begin to create a rhythm. It's almost as if you can't help yourself. Try it!

Music is used in meditation for a reason – it assists you in connecting to the higher vibrations where you can let go of the earthly ties and bring forth greater appreciation of what is good in your life. I must be clear that the music I am talking about is not about much of the music today where women are defiled by both men and women by name calling them "bitches" and worst, where anger and threats against others exist, and appreciation of life is scorned, and so much more. That music is abusive and offensive to all no matter where you are spiritually in life for it is the lowest form of negative vibration. It will hopefully one day be eliminated as we grow to love and respect each other in a greater way.

Prayer is one of the strongest ways to connect with your higher power – your own *personal* relationship with God. You don't need anyone else to pray for you (no one else has a greater power for you to connect with God than you do). However, praying in groups of two or more raises the vibrations so that the power of your prayer increases more than twofold each time another's prayer is added to the group. Group prayer is very powerful especially when healing another soul.

Yet oftentimes, we may pray to God to have him make a sick person well without taking into consideration that it may not be to their best interest to become well or it may not be part of their pre-life agreement where they agreed to experience what they are going through.

Rest assured that when you do pray to God, particularly with *gratitude*, you are heard. Yet again, we need to be reminded to pray so that we are not asking for more than what can be realistically given to us or what would be best for us. As a child, most don't understand the limitations of money as an obstacle to what they want. Although adults have a greater capability of looking at things differently and perhaps make their prayers more attainable, it does not mean that they should limit their requests as to whether they can afford it or not. If it is right for the request to be answered, it will be. Believe, trust, and accept the outcome as it is meant to be, knowing that God wants the best for us.

Prayer has power and if we use prayer in all the right ways, it is a magnificent means to increase our mass conscience energy in a positive way, which has the ability to overcome many issues and problems. Obviously, no prayers are answered that are requesting damage to another person or soul because God is love and wishes no harm to anyone or anything.

You can also pray and talk to your guides and angels, the Masters and anyone from the other side that you want to connect with – all prayers of love are welcomed.

Reading Spiritual Books is another great way to live in the higher mind. Reading the Bible and other like-minded books allows you to better appreciate yourself as a human being on the earth plane at this time with gratitude.

There is so much information available to us that we no longer have to be in the dark or without the tools that can elevate our spiritual sense and those energy vibrations, all of which bring us closer to our higher power. Reading is rewarding. There is *always* something new to be learned! Take the experiences and teachings from the books which resonate with you and leave the rest which is always personal for each of us.

All across our country, there are places that have different spiritual sessions available to you at a reasonable cost on many subjects. Take advantage of what is offered and learn, learn, learn to love and appreciate who **you** are!

Doing Something for Someone Else! is another simple way to raise your vibrations. When you do this, you automatically release yourself from the idea of coming from lack in any form and that you have more than enough to share with someone else whether it be money, love, time, energy or anything that can help another. Abundance is a high vibration.

It is important to stop complaining and gossiping because both of those frequencies are in the lower dimensions. Doing so is simply a waste of time with no true positive results. Remember the Law of Attraction? It is important to *expect* all the good in your life which *creates* the energy to have it.

Doing something positive that you have always wanted to do but have kept putting off, releases an exciting energy that can produce a positive perspective of "I can do anything I set my mind to do." You eliminate the fear to do it and expand the possibilities in life.

The most important things that you can do for you (and others) is to **Forgive** - forgive yourself and others. The act of forgiveness helps us to develop and nourish love in our lives because releasing blame and judgment of others, as well as ourselves, is imperative to succeed. And furthermore, when you let go of that blame and judgment of others you will find freedom to live your own life with greater acceptance of self. Forgiveness is humbling when we recognize and accept the idea that there really isn't right or wrong – only the truth of our beliefs - and for each of us that can be different. If we live listening to our inner voice that always guides us to higher living, forgiveness becomes easy. Holding onto anger, resentment, and judgment begins to become a heavy load of negative energy that doesn't serve us or others.

THANK YOU. LOVE YOU.

Love you, too.

Where there is love, there is healing.

Chapter 8

The God Energy and Why Am I Here?

The two most important days in your life are the day you are born and the day you find out why."

– Mark Twain

The more that I listened to all that "Jay" had to say, the more I needed to know about the God energy. Perhaps there is something within me that demands to know what is expected of me as an individual, and because we are all one, what is expected of us as a whole. When you look and see all the glory that is God in all the earth's beauty and the miracle of creation, it becomes obvious that we are more than just an occasional whim created by a higher energy – but to do what? How are we connected? What is our purpose here? Why would we chose to be here?

How often do we ask (and sometimes beg) God to help us in a particular situation and come to rely on Him for the answers to something as simple as whether to attend a certain gathering or not? We even turn to other modalities to bolster our own ideas and beliefs or sometimes to receive a clue as to the future without the prospective of inner thinking.

WHEN WE ASK GOD WHETHER TO ATTEND A PARTY OR NOT ETC., I BELIEVE THAT GOD ISN'T GOING TO BE BOTHERED WITH SOMETHING THAT TRIVIAL, AND ANY ANSWER REALLY COMES FROM OUR OWN SELF. IS THAT CORRECT?

In a sense that is correct. When you say that you believe that we get guidance from our self – of course we do. It is all one energy anyways. We split it up into other energies to help us understand it because it is different vibrational frequencies. But when we say that something comes through us, it is actually coming FROM us. Sometimes that is good and sometimes not so much.

BUT IS IT GOD SPEAKING TO US?

Sometimes. The way the vibrational frequencies are what you call God, the ultimate creative force, the thing that constantly churns out and creates and holds the space for all of creation, is an unbelievably high vibrational frequency. Most of us do not communicate directly with that frequency. However, we have to remember there are billions of tiny stepped-down frequencies of that. We can call them arch angels, masters, teachers, guides, whatever you want to call them. So wherever we are, whatever we have cleaned up, whatever filters are still running in there, we are going to be communicating with the closest vibrational frequency with God that we can or to the Godhead.

That means that if you are having a really bum day or someone hasn't cleaned out their stuff and they think that they are talking to God, well, they are in a sense, but it is not the pure, positive, creative force. It is a step-down version. And a lot of us fool ourselves into thinking it's that pure positive creative force because it just feels so good. When we get to those ever slightly step-down vibrations, they are just bliss – like the arch angels. We call them arch angels; we call them creations of God. They really are manifestations of specific characteristics of the creative force step-downed enough that they can interact with us directly. That is God interacting with us directly in a different way. So it is always us talking to self, I guess you would say. The only caution we get is that we are going to connect to whatever fits our vibrational frequencies. So are we talking to God? Yes.

The creative force is not the least bit concerned about things like deciding whether to attend a party. It doesn't even exist. It's the step-down versions, our own filters and understandings – all of that. But the godhead itself, no. It really doesn't care – it just holds that space for us.

Sometimes people get carried away. God told me this; God told me that. First off, sometimes it's a higher vibrational frequency and sometimes it's not. Sometimes it is just something that they wanted to do and they are doing it. So they heard what they wanted to hear. They also forget that God is not in the business of that. Creator is in the business of creating space for us so we can make our own choices, live our own lives, and evolve through our choices.

ONCE YOU START THINKING ABOUT IT THAT WAY, IT MAKES SUCH SENSE, DOESN'T IT?

Certainly.

IF YOU ARE TAKING DRUGS, YOU ARE RUNNING AWAY FROM LIFE OR TO FEEL GOOD. WHAT ARE SOME OF THE THINGS YOU CAN DO TO FEEL GOOD ON A DAILY BASIS AND MAKE YOU WANT TO LIVE WITHOUT DRUGS OR ADDICTION THAT ISN'T IN THE BOOK?

*Jay is saying that the entire book is about that and if you really want to summarize it, you can put it into the terms of this book gives a lot of starting points for anyone who knows they are dealing with addictions. It is important to look through it and see what is immediately applicable, what is available to them and to look at it NOT as something you HAVE TO do like going on a diet but to look at it as a **push for freedom, for power**. If they start on one thing and stay consistent with it, they are headed in the right direction, they are making progress. That is something people need to be aware of. Some people can jump in head first and they are going to be better off doing it all at once full force; other people are going to have to start with one thing, get good at it first, and then add on. So it is very individualized.*

JAY, DO YOU HAVE MORE HELPFUL TIDBITS?

I like that you helped that gal understand that she is not a failure for having an addiction. The only way we fail is if we stop trying and is something where we have been taught that addiction is a life-long battle. It does not have to be. It is not SUPPOSED to be.

If they realized that it is not going to be a struggle for the rest of their lives – all they have to do is take the first step with ABSOLUTE DETERMINATION. That's it. Determination to get your life back and those who don't want to, don't want to. Maybe not the best choice for them, but it's a choice and they don't have to.

One of the things I like about your books is that it helps the co-dependents begin to understand that they really cannot force change on the other person - it really is their responsibility to change themselves.

LOVE YOURSELF!

I WAS READING A PARTICULAR SPIRITUAL BOOK WHERE ONE OF HIS CLIENTS SUGGESTED THAT THE GOD ENERGY WAS THE BIG ENERGY, AND WE WERE THE ONES HAVING THE EXPERIENCES IN ORDER TO FEED THAT ENERGY TO GOD. THAT DOESN'T SOUND RIGHT TO ME. WHAT DO YOU THINK?

What he is saying is not true. He thinks that he has people who are coming from their higher self with no filter, but it is very clear from what this one is saying, he is coming from his own belief system. There is another point in that book where it states that God creates imperfect on purpose. That is just crap. We are created in perfection period. We are God expressing itself and experiencing life. That means that we are not forced to come here. It means that we are not made imperfect. We are expressions of God literally.

We are not off-shoots of God; we are God expressing itself and looking at the billions of unlimited opportunities for even greater understanding, and we get to choose which ones we want. We look at what we want and decide what is going to make us the most wonderful, great, glorious, all that good stuff, and we freely choose that. We are free to stop incarnating on this plane any time we want. He is putting forth a new version of the old God of being holy and mighty and we are at his mercy. and that is wrong – it is not the truth.

ALTHOUGH WE WORK ON THE OTHER SIDE FOR SPIRITUAL GROWTH, DOESN'T LIVING ON THE EARTH PLANE DEVELOP SPIRITUAL GROWTH QUICKER?

We keep calling it spiritual growth as expressions of God, but it is just experiencing life. Getting better and better at creating.

AND WE HAVE CHOICES OF WHERE TO GO, DON'T WE? THIS ISN'T THE ONLY PLACE WHERE OUR ENERGY CAN GO.

Exactly. He represents it as "Oh, poor us." We are going to go to school; we are going to get all this crap when we go back and say, "Wow! Screwed up that time." Or "Wow! Did really good in that one." We choose freely whether or not we are going to come back, what we want to work on, what we don't want to work on. We are not victims. It is actually a celebration!

JAY, HOW WOULD YOU DESCRIBE THE GOD ENERGY AND HOW WERE YOUR EXPERIENCES SO YOU NOW KNOW MORE AND MORE ABOUT THE GOD ENERGY?

Moving into what you are thinking of as the God energy is moving into a space of totality in the sense of I really and truly am everything. I am experiencing everything about life in every form, in every planet, every dimension – all one huge energy. I am IT. While I am it, I know that all of what I am doing is me. It is by my choice, free-will; it is an adventure. There is no such thing as "I am doing anything wrong" because I am just experiencing and creating. There may be times, for example, in the human form that what I am experiencing is less than perfect, when it is what you would call a wrong step, but even that is okay because I am absolutely, positively, sitting in the space of knowing that I am eternal, that I am perfection, that everything has reason, and that everything will work out just fine.

So it's not that I bury my head in the sand and say, Oh, gee, golly, that person is abusing that other person, but it will be fine, oh la la la. I see from the depths of my being in them why they are doing it and the incredible potential outcome and beyond that I know that everything is a state of perfection and MUST always return to that state of perfection. So I allow myself to play the game of not knowing myself and I monitor and watch and hold the space for all of this to happen.

Everything is actually in complete homeostasis. And I love. I love regardless of what any creature or human being or planet or asteroid is doing. It is life. All of life is sacred. And it is good. Now, that doesn't mean that I am going to sit back and not help those who are making choices that are hiding the perfection of life from themselves. And again, we have to use terminology where we are separate when we are really not. So I as a separate form that you would think of as Jay, I am going to get off my bum and do everything I can to help every person, place, thing, form, dimension, to remember the beauty that it really is. And it becomes a joyous celebration because what I am doing is bringing them back to exultation. Back to joy, love, laughter, freedom, everything. They literally are all that way. They just lost sight of it – that's all.

Love takes many forms. One form of the love is I AM the all-powerful, creative force creating and holding space – holding everything in the state of homeostasis. Even when you see wars breaking out on the planet such as yours, I am still holding everything in homeostasis so everyone can return. Another part of the love is I create forms, I love them, I nurture them. I am involved in their evolution because they are ME. And again, we are using terms of separation because our language at this time doesn't have anything else. But it's all ME. And you can say the same thing and the Arch Angels can say the same thing. The Masters have been telling us the same thing all this time now. We are all one. Now is ever-changing, ever-growing because of creation - that which is created must create. It is just life.

JAY, AFTER YOU PASSED CAN YOU DESCRIBE YOUR JOURNEY AND HOW YOU CONNECTED TO THE GOD ENERGY?

I did go through a progression. Remember your linear time - we can't even compare it to the reality of now. So, the progression I made here took place in what would have taken 10,000 years there - you would think of it as maybe a minute. And my progression was coming from the physical form into the realization of spiritual form; then, once I am in the realization of spiritual form, it is as if I reconnect with parts of who I am. It doesn't mean the soul has been segregated or separated; it means the memories, the greater memories of who I am, what I have been now become a normal part of what you would think of as my consciousness. Then I go forward in my spiritual understanding of love – of why we are doing what we are doing, reconnecting.

Now a part of that is what I am doing with you. It is moving through – creating a greater understanding – and in doing this, I create some greater understanding for myself and reverse some of the not-so-positive effects of what happened when I was here on earth. And again, I am using terms of separation because we don't have anything else. I always try to think of it as going back to the Source – the All That Is – like you said, the All. Then, as I am progressing forward, I become more and more aware of – there you think of it as the ones in higher spaces, the old ones, the Ascended Masters, the Arch Angels – here we know it as those bits of God that have already experienced a lot more than I have. As I move more and more into that level, I am able to move further into the knowing of Source.

But when we cross over, depending on the individual, of course, it is different for everyone, but the general theme that is always the same, if you go wherever you want to go, you go to whatever you believe in because mind and emotions are the physical aspects of the creative intelligence. If you have used your mind and emotions while in the physical body to create a specific world – say for example, someone who is paranoid who says that everyone is out to get me, it's not my fault, dog eat dog, etc. – you have created that reality for yourself. So if you stay that way, you will go to that reality first.

But you have so much help to come out of it. You can be there a second or you can be there a lot longer. But again, that is choice of creation. You are not forced to go there. If someone has a wake-up call at the last minute, they don't need to go there at all. They can go to a higher realm – a different realm. So for every single person, what you are creating as the essence of who you are is where you will go when you cross over. It is a vibrational link.

Most of the people on the planet right now will go to a nice place that is peaceful and calm; it is loving; there is a lot of laughter; it is not what you think of as the highest realm, but it is spiritual home that is very nurturing, loving and helps us to progress and clear up whatever misunderstanding that we have created in our energy and move forward from there. It is very much like classrooms in the sense you were talking about before in that book, but it is joyful and not nearly as segregated as given in the book. There are moments when we will go into small study groups, of course, and regularly, but most of what we do is done in joyous love and celebration even when we don't do so great in our lifetimes. We still have the joy and loving support that we need. And so, I went through a progression of that.

AT ONE POINT, JAY, YOU SAID THAT A MASTER WOULD LOWER HIS VIBRATION AND HELP RAISE YOURS TO GO TO A HIGHER DIMENSION AND THAT IT WAS JESUS.

That is the one I knew and I called on so he is the one that met me. When you think of the Master who reaches forward to bring you up to a higher level, when we speak of it in earth terms, it is as if someone who is of greater wisdom reaches down, lifts, raises the vibrations, etc. To a degree that is true. But also in that process that would take 10,000 years there and you might think of it as a split second over here, it is me opening myself up to greater learning to working, studying, playing, laughing, and remembering. It is me doing my part so that I can also stretch up to meet that higher vibrational frequency. We all have that assistance. We all have energies that are more highly developed aspects of God than we are, reaching down to help us while we reach up – always forever – no matter what your form – whether you are in spirit or non-spirit. It doesn't matter.

So when I am speaking of the Master who helped me up, yes, Jesus is my chosen teacher and mentor. I will study more closely with others who are under him, but I also work with him. The way that we think of it now in earth terms is of a hierarchal structure. It is similar to that. It is just that what we call the hierarchal structure here there is absolutely zero judgment of better or worse. Remember when Jesus was on the earth plane and he said, "This that I do, you shall do and more." He said that because we believed we were less than, but in his eyes we are equal. And that is true of every higher being. Every higher expression of God believes that we who consider ourselves lower are equals. We just haven't discovered it yet. The only judgment comes from us. When we look at it as OOPS, screwed that up.

Jay, soul groups on the other side — do we continue to be in the same soul groups throughout our lifetimes?

To a large degree. Think of it like any kind of a school room. Some individuals in a specific class will be gifted in one area, some in another, some won't show any specific inclination toward any special area. The same thing happens in our soul experience. We will stick mainly with the main soul groups, but sometimes one will move far ahead, and another time one will kind of lag behind or choose a different area of specialization, based upon what they feel they need or want.

So soul groups are not poured into cement. They usually stay together, but there is a flexibility in there that is very noticeable. Say for example, a member of a soul group advances to the point where their experience of life (again we have to use subjective terms) is greater than the rest of the soul group. That member may or may not continue lessons the same way as the others although he can still interact any time. He quite often will interact with individuals in physical form as a way of assisting them to connect with that higher vibrational frequency to make different choices.

So, yes. Soul groups can number in the hundreds of thousands. They can be very small or they can be huge. There can be soul groups within soul groups. Think of it like a high school. Say you have seniors in high school.

There is a group for drama, there is a group for basketball; there is a group for football; there is a group for debate; there is a group for chess, etc. Soul groups are that way, too, in their interests and in their personalities. The part that book is talking about - first it is filtered through the belief systems that are prevalent on the earth plane right now. The second is it looks at it as if each individual is less than. The very premise of being created imperfect completely destroys the idea of Oneness. So it is quite different here, but it is wonderful. At the very least, most of the population will pass into a level of spirit where they feel peace and hope. That's the least for the average person!

THERE ARE A LOT OF PEOPLE, PARTICULARLY THE YOUNG, WHO ARE DYING AND CROSSING BECAUSE OF DRUGS AND ALCOHOL.

Yes. We do the best we can to assist them. Some of these individuals came in with a plan to leave early, but did not plan to do so through drug abuse. They got tied up in the static vibrational frequencies. Part of what has happened in the earth plane is the basic physical DNA has been mutated. It is reacting or mutated from the incredibly static energy that we have been generating there for a long time. The static energy doesn't just come from technology – it comes from all the negative thoughts, emotions, the wars, the hatred, the vendettas, all of these things that we have created, and some of these souls coming in are individuals who had hoped to use this time of rapid change to make different choices in how they handle life and don't handle life. You have a very, mixed bag of young people there right now. Some of them are individuals who have never, ever used drugs before, but they bow to peer pressure.

There is a book by Malcom Gladwell where he talks about the tipping point that refers to the monkeys on the island where the one monkey washed his sweet potatoes in the water. None of the others did and he was ostracized. Then, a couple more monkeys joined him, then, a couple more joined them, etc. until at one time at a very specific point enough monkeys started washing their sweet potatoes that the entire population of monkeys on that island automatically started washing their sweet potatoes. And it was discovered that the other monkeys being studied on other islands who had not started it at the same point the rest of the monkeys started on that first island, all of the other monkeys on the other islands started. What we are dealing with here now is that same phenomenon with human beings with self-destruction. You see it in things like Sandy Hook where kids go shooting up schools; you see it in kids committing suicide deliberately; you see it in kids giving into the addictions. We have reached a tipping point and it is now in epidemic proportion for that energy and the children are in the epidemic. And now it has become so acceptable and so common that it is presented to every single child. And if they have any kind of pattern of victim consciousness or entitlement or resentment or any former addictions they are extremely vulnerable to it.

Many of the kids who are dying from substance abuse came in to try and help change that. And, of course, we always make gold out of straw – if one crosses early, whether it is an accidental overdose or suicide, everything possible is done to create a ripple effect that will assist others to use it as a lesson. The problem is because it is so prevalent now, it is often seen as, "Well, they do it, it is okay. I can do it, too." Self-destruction is in epidemic proportion here right now.

So what are the things to do to help with that? Obviously, we are getting help from the other dimensions, what do we do here?

If each individual would be careful to monitor their thoughts, keep them in power, rather than powerless, it would make a huge difference. It is also moving out of the state of being afraid to hurt someone's feelings. We have gone from "It's okay to hurt someone's feelings" and being quite brutal about it in the past to "My goodness. We don't want to hurt their little soul; let's just give them whatever they want." We have to find a middle ground where we can use what we call tough love. Tough love isn't actually tough; it is common sense. It is survival. Not being able to use tough love with children is an insecurity in the parents. There needs to be a movement among parents and educators, who will stand up and say, "NO, it is not okay. These are the immediate consequences if you do that." There also needs to be a stand up in government – in all government organizations because right now they are very ineffectual.

MANY OF THE GOVERNMENT PROGRAMS DON'T ALLOW KIDS TO BE IN THERAPY OR REHAB LONG ENOUGH.

That is part of the problem, but it is a problem created by the initial problem. The initial one is that drugs are readily available; there are minimum consequences for the young people who do drugs. The problem is not with the rehab system – it is with the system that allows this to happen in the first place. That's parents, organizations, governments - it is the entire mentality. So if we really want to create a change, it has to come from the generations that are supposed to be assisting the children.

YOU COME TO THE POINT WHERE YOU HAVE NO CONTROL OVER THE OTHER PERSON AND YOU CAN'T FORCE THEM TO CHANGE.

That's right. That is why it must be done when they are young. They must receive the assistance when they are young. Then once you reach the point where you no longer have control over them, you do have control over them. Many of the parents there now continue to take care of their children because their children no longer care for themselves due to their substance abuse. They don't want to take responsibility for their own lives. The parent is afraid they are going to be living on the street, they are going to hit rock bottom, they are going to kill themselves, they are going to do whatever it is and because the parent lives in fear, the child stays in addiction. It is the parent's fear that needs to be healed too.

I BELIEVE THAT SOMETIMES (AND I DID THIS SOMETIMES WITH JAY) THAT I WOULD RATHER HAVE HIM LIVE IN THE HOUSE, BE ABLE TO TALK TO HIM, BE ABLE TO TELL HIM THAT I LOVE HIM, THAT I DON'T LIKE HIS BEHAVIOR OR AGREE WITH IT THAN HAVE HIM OUT ON THE STREET WHERE HE CAN HURT SOMEONE ELSE OR GET HURT.

But you are condoning the behavior by setting up a situation allowing him to continue. That is why it is so tough on parents. You have to take that chance – you would look at it as a choice of two evils. But the parents who allow the child to be self-destructive, and we'll talk about you and me specifically, Mom, but this is in general. The parents who allow the child to remain in self-destructive behavior because they are afraid it might get worse if they take steps to help are not helping – they are living in fear and enabling the child to stay exactly the way he or she is. Now, in this case, when it gets to the point that it is so bad, you are right, the rehab programs are not sufficient. But again, we have to go to resources, to parent responsibility.

Now, Mom, about you and me. When I was growing up there weren't a lot of resources. There was nobody to say, "Hey, this is what is going on. This is what is causing it; this is what we need to do to fix it, etc." So we had to just do the best that we could. That is not true anymore. Parents DO have resources to fix themselves and to help fix their children. They absolutely do. A lot of them are afraid to do it because they are afraid their child won't love them anymore. They are willing to risk the child wasting its entire life because they don't want to feel the child doesn't like them. That's a problem.

When you and I were going through it, again, we didn't have the resources that are available now, but your decisions were not based on will he love me, will he not love me, that wasn't a question. The question was how do I keep him from creating more harm to himself and to others?

THAT'S TRUE.

So we have a little bit of comparing apples to oranges and bananas here. But right now, the parents who say I am so afraid that he will never speak to me again, afraid that he will go live on the streets, etc. are doing great harm to their children. And their children are doing great harm to them!

WELL, I CAN REMEMBER HAVING JAY IN THERAPY AND HAVING HIM TESTED AND NOBODY KNEW WHAT WAS GOING ON WITH HIM.

Exactly. And I didn't know. There were no resources. If you were lucky enough to stumble on someone – ½ of a ½ of a ½ of the population knew about this stuff. And, of course, there was no world-wide web, no easy access to information. But parents cannot use that excuse anymore, and we don't mean to be harsh on them here. And I certainly don't because of what you and I went through. But there is no excuse for saying I can't do anything – I have no power.

OKAY, GOT IT.

At the very least, they could create rules in the house for the child, making them responsible for him or herself, and stick to it. That is one of the key problems. So many parents will move in the right direction, but then the child says, "Well, I am going to kill myself; I am going to live on the street; you don't love me anymore; don't you want to help me?" and the parents buy into it. We are not saying that it is the parent's fault (it takes two to create a mess; actually, it has taken many millions to create a mess like this) but it is a recurring cycle and both are locked in. The one who is not in the substance abuse has the greater burden of seeing the truth and acting on it. They both bear the burden or bear the responsibility. The substance abuse is really the out-picturing of all of the anger, fear, rage, release systems, blah, blah, that have been prevalent here for so long.

ISN'T IT TRUE THAT MANY OF US HAVE CHOSEN TO BE HERE TOGETHER BECAUSE WE BELIEVED THAT WE HAD A GREATER CHANCE OF RAISING THE VIBRATION?

Absolutely. We always bring our support system with us. And others of our soul group we bring together because we know that they are going to bring everything to the surface. Oftentimes, your worst enemy is one of your best friends on the other side. People would be surprised how often that happens.

EXPLAIN THAT PLEASE.

Our best friends hold the mirror up for us. It is a chance for accelerated rate of progression, accelerated difference in choices. And if you don't want to see that, we will perceive it as our enemy. And lots of times, they will come in, for example, in toxic relationships. If we have a toxic pattern that we have decided that we are by golly going to make different choices this time, we will very likely draw in someone who will complement that by keeping us in that pattern. We hope that we are going to do it a different way, but frequently we don't.

YEAH, I CAN VOUCH FOR THAT.

So you really don't know who the member of your soul group is by whether or not you like them. You don't have to like them, but you sure can learn from them. Then you can love them.

WE SURE DO ALL HAVE OUR JOURNEYS, DON'T WE?

Yes, and when we make the plans, we specifically set it up to make other choices. Do we plan to suffer? No, we do not. Our entire purpose is to make choices that create paradise. We have the contingencies for suffering in there because we know that we are not going to make all the right choices. We are just creating suffering that way. We never, ever deliberately choose a life of suffering saying, "Well, I am going to suffer through the whole thing, and then I will be okay." We may choose a life of what we would call suffering here thinking. "Good, I will rise above it and have a beautiful life."

So when your friend says, "why would anyone choose this?" That is a loaded question. This that she is perceiving is not what we are choosing or not what we chose when we incarnated. It is what we are creating as we go along. We chose a life of overcoming and triumphing, and we put everything in place to do that, but we keep making the same ole choices that created a mess in the first place. Every time we make a different choice, we are actually choosing in accordance with our plan. So she asked more questions than she realized. We did not choose the results that we are seeing. Oops!

JAY, DO YOU HAVE ANYTHING ELSE TO ADD?

Yes. This whole issue of free will – it is extremely important for people to understand, particularly with regard to addiction. When you see someone who is addicted, it looks as if they have no choice. And frequently, when they are locked into whatever their thought and emotional pattern is, they have put themselves in a position not of no choice, but of being locked into choosing badly, and being locked into thinking they can't help it. Free will exists period. It is there for us at all times. If we bury it deep enough, it is harder to get to, that's all, or it's harder to realize that it is there for us at all times. If we bury it deep enough, it is harder to get to, or it's harder to realize.

That might help a lot of parents when they see their beloved children going through what they think of as hell, and creating their own hell as well. To realize that they absolutely do have the free will and ability to come out of that at any time, but they are not going to do it as long as they are allowed to stay in it. As long as they are comfortable and getting their basic needs met, they are going to keep making the same choices.

And when you talk about energy and the Oneness and the All, even that energy we are talking about that is the addict who appears to have no free will, is the energy of the All. It is the one that is experiencing what it feels like to be powerless, angry or frustrated. And basically, substance abuse is trying to return to how we feel in spirit by false means. And sometimes, it is just trying to escape the responsibilities we have created for ourselves. So there are a lot of things behind substance abuse and the reason people go into it.

The fact is yes, all of life is created in perfection. We have the free will to create ourselves as always reflecting that perfection, always being that perfection or not. There are life forms that have chosen differently - not to the point where you would think of them as actually evil. It does exist. It's the minority, but it does exist. And every now and then, you will run into one there on the earth plane. *You call them sociopaths. Now some of those whom you would call sociopaths are just expressions of God who have gotten very lost. They will come back again. But there is that rare occasion where it is one who will NOT come back willingly. That one will be re-absorbed, not in the sense of losing individual identity, but in the sense of being allowed to start from a clean slate because there is no chance of it making choices that will allow it to bring itself back. Nothing is ever left out; even the most heinous or what you would think of as evil person will always be brought back to love. We will never, ever abandon any life form, ever.*

We are careful about spreading this information because so many people will jump onto the band wagon and will become so dramatic, "Oh well, that one is an evil soul," or "That one is going to have to be re-done," or "It's not my fault – the person I am dealing with chose evil." They use it to dodge responsibility instead of using information like discernment. But for the sake of your understanding in this information that you are bringing through, we bring this through to you.

THANK YOU.

It is especially important to say that no creation will ever be left out of love, for any reason. It may bring itself back or we will assist in bringing it back or we will assist those that will come; we will simply bring it back if it does not chose to do so. Sometimes that takes a very, very, long time for the ones who have gone that far. But it will happen. Nothing is ever left out of love because it is all the One – it is all ME as I am. Everything is precious. So it is extremely important for individuals reading your book that they have an understanding of who they really are and the role each plays. It is about them moving from a space of powerless and looking at the addicts as helpless to the space of pure power and assisting others to realize their power. That's all.

The fact that you choose to come here when it is not really a picnic at all tells you how powerful you are as souls. In the power of form as your soul, you can do this, and you can, and you will - we just have to lighten up.

Just by being here is a glorious choice that we actually work very hard to earn. In the spiritual world, earn is a joy, a celebration. It's a, "I deserve this. I am wonderful." We earn it from the other side. We have the privilege of coming here.

JAY, DO YOU HAVE ANYTHING ELSE TO ADD?

We are not going to cross over and be made to feel bad and hate ourselves and all that. It is one of the problems with some books that have that judgment in it. It makes us dread crossing over when there is really nothing to dread . . . Only love awaiting us.

I LOVE YOU, JAY PECK.

Love you ... always and forever.

Where there is love, there is healing.

I Know This to Be True

I realize that I was blessed in that Jay and I were open enough to discuss addiction, some of his actions, dreams, and philosophies about spirituality and life, and some of mine. We both were very aware of the hole he was in with his addiction and the improbability of his walking away from addiction this lifetime. And knowing that and living those last two years before his death were painful for both of us beyond anything I can express. Yet, at the time of his death, there was JOY, as weird as that sounds. I no longer had to worry whether he was okay or safe, that he hadn't been physically hurt by others or that he hadn't hurt anyone as sometimes can happen under the influence of drugs and alcohol. Instead, I was surrounded by such JOY knowing that Jay would be in a place surrounded by unconditional love and no longer in pain. It was important for me to know he would be surrounded by others who would comfort him and love him because, as his mother, I am sure you can understand and possibly relate to that.

But the biggest JOY comes as I am communicating with him while writing our books or just sharing thoughts. I am very aware of our pre-life contract and feel again so blessed to have experienced and share what we have learned about addiction, painful as it was at times. We are grateful if what we share can give guidance, understanding, love and peace to anyone. It is time for us as a society to address addiction in new and different ways as there is so much joy ahead for all of us if we are open to it and allow it in.

Although it may seem as if I breezed through Jay's death, feeling relieved that he was no longer in physical and emotional pain, and feeling great joy in his being surrounded by unconditional love, I still had my moments. Moments of sadness, of questioning, of feeling guilty, of anger, and most importantly, moments of hope when I began communicating with him shortly after his death.

We often overlook many daily messages and signs from our loved ones from the other side and, instead, long for more "in your face" physical signs to prove that our loved one is with us. I am no different for at times that is exactly what I wanted and needed after Jay died. I have been fortunate to experience a few of those "in your face" happenings that I share with you that confirms for me what Jay said ("We don't die!"). I hold that statement to be true.

In springtime 2006, a few months after his death, I was having a lonely day, feeling the loss of Jay. As soon as I woke up that morning, I was insistent that he give me a physical sign to show that he was okay, still loved me and was near.

I gathered Sweet Pea, my puppy, for her early morning walk, taking the same route as we did each day, walking along the street that encircles our little community. We had not gone far when she stopped, and I looked down to see a gold and diamond heart pendant laying in the road. An odd peace came over me and I just knew that Jay had sent it. I was ecstatic and filled with humor for Jay knew this would be the perfect token of his love because I love anything glitzy! Particularly if it is a good piece of jewelry.

However, as we humans often do, I began to doubt and question whether this was indeed from Jay. So I called the guard at the gate of our development, asking if anyone had reported a missing piece of jewelry. No one had. I left my name at the gate in case anyone did. No one ever did. Several days went by with no word of anyone losing jewelry. Finally, I asked Jay if he had sent this to me. He laughed and said he had. I treasure it.

Another time, in the summer of that year, I was missing Jay - though I was not sad or upset – just missing him. I was standing near the pool at dusk watching it grow dark when all of a sudden a bright light, looking much like lightning, flashed through the center of the pool from one end to another. Again, an odd peace overcame me and I thought how beautiful. I didn't think about it again until Jay asked me how I liked it, that it was he who had done that. Another wonderful sign that he is always near.

The following spring, a dear friend came to stay with me for several months. She, along with her children, had been part of the Christmas holiday time with Jay and me for several years. She was devastated by his death, and talked about him a lot during her visit. Not surprising, we always seemed to see hawks circling which is the animal spirit symbol for him, and I knew that he was around.

One day, she and I were off to visit our mutual friend across town and were waiting at a stop light at one of the larger intersections not far from our friend's house. The light changed, and we were first in the left lane about to turn when a car came barreling through the intersection, out of control, headed our way. My friend began screaming, "Oh my God! They are going to hit us!"

And I thought so, too. The cars were facing each other front end to front end. I could see the expressions of terror on their faces inside the car when all of a sudden we watched their car literally pushed away from us. It was the oddest sensation because there is no way any car is able to do that. The car was tipped up on two wheels moving not forward but sideways. We escaped that accident but I knew deep in my heart that Jay had something to do with it. When I asked him, he said, "I was a part of it, but it took five of us to do that."

When I asked him who was involved, he said, "Part of the group."

I am not unique in receiving help and messages from the other side from so many who are waiting to be noticed. We all receive them, we just need to be aware of our surroundings and the people who we are in contact with each day for they are often the ones who unwittingly hold our message.

It is so comforting to know that we are always loved and are often shown that love from those souls on the other side, our own cheering squad, if you will. And the best news is that each of us has one.

Jay says: *so, dear reader, know that we don't die — we continue to grow, learn and love on the other side as you do there, and we carry that into each lifetime we experience. We share our wisdom with the living in many ways — small and more noticeable. All you have to do is be open to receive them.*

Remember, too, how powerful you are to make the choices you need to in order to live in the higher-minded ways — the beautiful ways of living without addiction. We are all cheering you on — believe it, know it — you can do it!

I love you, Jay Peck! I am honored to have been your mother this lifetime, and love you more than words can express. I am grateful for our life together with all of its experiences that has provided both of us spiritual growth. For that, I am blessed. You are part of my heart forever.

Namaste, dear one.